NUR-E-AMBER

A Journey of Healing, Transformation and Rebirth

Amber Khan

Amber Khan

Introducing the **7 Zones** to Heal & transform

your mind, body & soul,

The **GAIA Diet**, The **Two Golden Hours** of the Day & the **Glide Vantage**

Align to your source, find your purpose & unveil the power of your subconscious mind.

First Edition Drafted March 7, 2020

First Edition Published April 13, 2020

☐

Nur-e-Amber

Amber Khan

Copyright © 2020 by Amber Khan

ISBN:

979-8642240557

—

Book Cover Copyrights

Amber Khan

Contents

Nur e Amber

The essence of healing & transformation.

You are a 'Timeless soul' in a 'Timed world'

The idea is to live through this world with the physical body but not any attachment. You are an eternal being passing through this 'Earth'. Experience, learn, and 'Glide' through life and be so liberated that nothing controls you. You are not here to suffer, you are here to flow, learn, create, ascend, assist, and connect to your source.

When you trust the 'Divine Intelligence' for guidance and direction, you automatically choose the highest outcome. When you make a choice yourself, you override the divine wisdom as it doesn't have power over your choice. It guides you but ultimately your choice determines the outcome. The idea is not to 'Achieve' but 'Align'. Once you align, everything will automatically fall into place bringing you peace, serenity, abundance, and success.

Align, Ask & Allow

Sometimes we are taken away from what we think is our life and redirected to a life that we are meant to have; leading to our purpose. We should consider ourselves lucky if this happens. Not everyone is lucky to get this personal attention from the divine power; you are. In all chaos and disorder; there is always a secret and an order. What seems like chaos to you is an orchestrated and orderly chain of events by the universe. It's the rearrangement and redirection.

There is nothing in this universe that you can't achieve, do, or allow in your experience. Return to who you were meant to be. Realign with your 'Source', the 'Universe', 'Earth energy. Every soul who has chosen to let go of a negative state and rise up to rebirth, has found everything they have ever dreamt of as the rising soul from the darkness to light always has more courage, strength, faith, passion, humbleness, and more will-power; that ultimately sculpts their life exactly how they desire.

We can let this negative overpower our entire being or we can take the reins back in our hands and turn this negative into the biggest positive for us. We can't undo what happened but we can outdo our current state and choose to live the best life possible. We have the power of choice.

Allow yourself to activate the deep intense soul fulfilling love that is in your own soul. You are who you have been waiting for; it is your own love that you seek. When you begin to truly love yourself and remember how extraordinary you truly are, you will connect and merge into the divine sacred source's love.

Welcome

Welcome to this, 'Earth Life Dimension'. You are the universe within, powerful beyond words, thoughts, and vibrations. You are here for a purpose and you will leave this dimension once your purpose is achieved. Your 'Avatar' is to find yourself; sync with your ultimate source, align with the infinite wisdom, and to connect your vibrations back to your destiny.

You will experience magnificence and more during this journey. You will learn lessons and mold your daily life accordingly. The life that you have experienced until now is the past, which is also an illusion. The life's moments that you are experiencing presently and the ones coming will transform as you will be guided towards your purpose. Your journey inwards will unveil the magnificent powers that link you to the ultimate energy and destination; your purpose.

Get ready to be aligned; to your source.

***

Part 1

The Incident

"Life has many ways of testing a person's will, either by having nothing happen at all or by having everything happen all at once."

—Paulo Coelho

August 2012

Seeing my husband's face at the airport, I felt a warm feeling rush over me, and the same thought came to my mind once again; maybe things could work out. After 13 years of a marriage filled with pain, suffering, loneliness, and eventually a mental separation, today again in my optimistic attitude and hope, it felt like it may work.

We went home and it was strangely beautiful or maybe it was just home. It felt calm and serene, I felt like I belonged there or maybe I was being too optimistic. 16 hours later came an argument, followed by another and then the brutal realization that it would always be like this and then the unthinkable happened;

He hit me, again & again, brutally.

Everything just halted inside me, my emotions, my senses, my tears, my fears; in that moment my entire world collapsed. I lost my hope, my home, my partner, my security, my faith, my marriage, my trust, my positivity, me; my whole life changed in front of my eyes as I passed out on the floor.

"Walking away from someone who hurts you isn't an act of negativity towards them. It's an act of positivity towards yourself."

—Anonymous

Sitting at the same airport again, my heart ached, I was leaving my world. I was in a complete state of shock. Feeling numb and lifeless, I couldn't feel or hear the external world. All I could see was the crashing of an entire life. My feet felt so heavy; every step was painful. I walked towards the plane feeling a rush to turn back and go, but where and to whom. I didn't want to leave, but in that moment, I had no other choice.

The 'Now' felt like the most painful moment. The past had thrown me out and the future was not visible. Left in the present, which was painful, lonely, bitter, and very scary, I walked to my seat and sat down. Tears were flowing down my face, and I felt like the weakest person. I had no strength to feel anything anymore, I closed my eyes trying to make the 'Now' disappear. I went into the past and didn't want to come back. I thought about the few beautiful times and the thoughts moved towards the events that were painful and bitter. I still didn't open my eyes; it was easier to stay in the pain. I was too scared to open my eyes to enter the present.

After a very long flight to the other side of the world, during which I cried all the way, I was back in Arizona; I felt dead. I could see my parents standing and waiting for me. From afar, I could see the pain in my father's eyes; the tears that he was trying to hold. I wish I could change that moment. They were hurt because I was hurt. They were in pain because I was in pain.

Going back to my parents' home after 13 years felt like I had failed.

Over the next few days, I fell into a deep depression and was miserable. Nothing kept my mind away from the agony and misery. I stared at the ceiling for hours and hours, sometimes days, and asked the question, 'Why?' My body was bruised badly but my soul was hurting more than the physical bruises. He had attacked my soul; my optimism and my trust.

I had tried everything in my power to make this marriage work. Where did I go wrong? What could I have done better? How could I have made things work? Through all these thoughts I realized that it wasn't me. He didn't want this as he had other plans. He didn't want me in his life anymore and he made me leave. This thought made me realize that it wasn't my fault! I fell prey to his scheme of having me leave. It wasn't my fault; what a powerful thought. IT WASN'T MY FAULT!

After the incident, I kept wondering, how could a man do this to the woman he claimed to love, to the woman he had promised to protect, to the woman who was the mother of his children, to the woman who had supported him in his struggles and dreams, but more so to the woman he claimed to love.

Throughout the 13 years, I knew that the river that I was flowing in was not meant for me. I tried to swim out of it several times but couldn't. I felt helpless, trapped, and miserable. Sometimes I got to the shore but swam back because I was too scared to start my journey back on land; in the land of the unknown. This immensely negative event in my life was actually a blessing in disguise. The river that I was trying to get out from had hit a cliff and the water had thrown me out with a very strong blow. It was painful but it was a blessing; a realization that came to me in the following years as everything unfolded in my life.

"Pain doesn't show up in our lives for no reason. It's a sign that something in our lives need to change."

—Mandy Hale

As we go on our journey through life our mind helps us make decisions but mostly our heart leads in answering our puzzles; we just don't pay attention to it. We focus more on the mind and think that it's right. We should listen to our heart, our intuition, and our gut. There is a reason it speaks. It works with our subconscious. Our mind focuses on the present but our subconscious analyzes the future. We fail to recognize and act on it. We should; our heart guides us better.

"In all chaos there is a cosmos, in all disorder a secret order."

—Carl Jung

If an event, an individual, or a scenario is causing us pain, then there is a reason behind it. It's a sign that something is not aligned. We should not overlook that pain because eventually it will come out in one way or another; maybe at a time when we are least prepared for it.

This Incident was my redirection.

Healing Begins

So, how did I heal? How can you heal?

Healing Therapies to get through life's difficult moments

Acceptance

Accept what has happened! You don't need to know and figure out the reason for now. Just accept and process it. It is one of the most painful acts but acceptance starts the healing process. Personally, it took me a long time to accept, but once I did, I started to heal. Though it is rough, you have to leave the victim mindset because otherwise, it will poison you completely. You will feel depressed and weak but you are going to have to try to move past this.

"Ruin is a gift. Ruin is the road to transformation."

—Elizabeth Gilbert (Eat Pray Love)

Everything happens for a reason. You will get to know your reason along the journey. For now, focus on the first step, come out of the shock that your mind and body are in. Breathe, relax, and accept the situation. There is a reason why it happened, and you don't know it yet, but you will. Life has its ways of testing you. Life is unpredictable. We go through each day of our lives taking every person, moment, and thing for granted, as this is human nature. We are never prepared for the worst but we are always excited for the best and willingly accept all the best with open arms.

Accept your history and the people that have been a part of your history; accept your circumstances and remember that none of these define you. Acceptance is the first step to letting go and setting yourself free. Carrying bitterness, anger or animosity burdens no one but you.

Acceptance of the worst eases you from inside. You don't have to accept it as if you deserved it. You have to accept it as a life event. From this moment on, you will be a different person & your life will be different. You will learn from this and face things differently. You will come out of your dreamland and face reality. You will make better decisions in the future.

Let go!

"Two monks were on a pilgrimage. One day, they came to a deep river. At the edge of the river, a young woman sat weeping because she was afraid to cross the river without help. She begged the two monks to help her. The younger monk turned his back. The members of their order were forbidden to touch a woman.

But the older monk picked up the woman without a word and carried her across the river. He put her down on the far side and continued his journey. The younger monk came after him, scolding him and berating him for breaking his vows. He went on this way for a long time. Finally, at the end of the day the older monk turned to the younger one. "I only carried her across the river. You have been carrying her all day."

—Zen Tale

Letting go can be difficult. Letting go of people, ideas, expectations, and desires. Letting go of bad habits, false beliefs, and unhealthy relationships... the list goes on. Every day, every moment presents an opportunity to create ourselves anew, to shrug off the baggage of the past, open ourselves up to the possibility of the moment and take action to create an incredible future.

Although we can understand this intellectually, knowing it and living it are two very different things.

Believe in yourself. Believe in your purpose.

Every single soul in this universe is here for a reason. There is no individual that does not have a purpose or duty. We are all here to love and be loved. We are here to serve and be served. We are here to cherish and be cherished. We have to believe in this and find our divine purpose.

Sometimes we are taken away from what we think is our life to a life that we are meant to have. We should consider ourselves lucky if this happens. Not everyone is lucky to get this personal attention from the divine power. You are!

That's the reason you're directed now. It's time for you to go to your path, to your journey, to what you are meant to be. I believe the universe always has plans beyond our perception. Sometimes things don't go our way, but trust in the bigger picture, and know there is a reason and a lesson. You may not realize it today or even years down the road, but there is one.

"Believe that the universe is unfolding as it should and that you have a divine role to play. Believe that holding on does nothing in fact but hold you back from that purpose."

—Karine Chalmers

Surrender

Imagine yourself swimming in the ocean. Feel the water and the beautiful sun. Feel the powerful waves and the smoothness of the current taking your body with its gentle strength. Now try swimming against it. Try fighting the tide and going against the gentleness of water. Suddenly it will become the most powerful enemy. Stop now; stop going against the tide.

Surrender yourself; don't resist it. It will exhaust and drain you and eventually win; just go with the flow. Close your eyes and believe in the power that is directing you. Believe that it is a rearrangement & a redirection. Just close your eyes, lower your head, ease your shoulders, relax your body, and release your soul from this pain & surrender. Things will start working out after this moment as you're not fighting things anymore. Once you stop resisting them, they will start working in your favor.

"Try not to resist the changes that come your way. Instead let life move through you. And do not worry that your life is turning upside down. How do you know that the side you are used to is better than the one to come?"

—Mevlana Rumi

Analysis

Take time to reflect on your own history like a third party without judgment. Understand that you are not your past. Understand that the situations, patterns, and people in your life created your experiences. Knowing and understanding your past and some of your patterns will help you recognize why you hold on and repeat certain behaviors.

Understanding creates awareness; awareness helps you break the cycle.

Sit back, take a deep breath, and reflect on your life and the recent experiences. Why did all this happen? What was your role in it? What could you have done to avoid it? What was the communication gap? Analyze one incident at a time and see where you went wrong. Maybe you didn't but maybe you did. Could you have avoided the argument or reaction by doing things differently? Taking time to analyze yourself because it makes it easier for you to understand yourself. This is needed so that you don't repeat behaviors, actions, or reactions in the future.

The way we respond when things don't go our way is where the power lies. Our attitude to handle this moment is our test; choosing to react or respond is the key to the results. I believe that things usually seem worse right in that moment. We are too caught up emotionally to be objective; we may have unrealistic expectations, or we try to take too much control of things. We build stories in our mind, and they can sometimes spiral out of control. We get into the over-thinking mode and it's like quicksand. It sucks you in and keeps descending you and you lose control. Train your mind to become aware of this mode and save yourself from it as it initiates. Put yourself in the other person's shoes and try to understand the source of their pain. This surely requires a very compassionate heart but this ritual will ease your heart.

Gratitude

This is truly a miracle prayer: gratitude. When life takes you to the hardest point, give thanks for the good that you have. Close your eyes and think about all the good things you're thankful for; your health, your kids, your parents, your friends, your work, your achievements, your accomplishments, and much more. We all have different things in life to be thankful for. Make a list and read it over and over again. It will make you smile and it will let the universe know you're happy and you'll be returned with more things to be thankful for. This is a simple secret!

"Gratitude is a powerful process for shifting your energy and bringing more of what you want in life. Be grateful for what you already have and you will attract more good things."

—Rhonda Byrne (The Secret)

Accepting or not accepting the Gift

A Wonderful Story Attributed to Buddha

"Once Buddha was travelling in the company of several other people. One of the travelers begins to test Buddha by responding to anything he had

to say with disparaging, insulting, hurtful remarks. Every day for the next three days, this traveler just verbally abused Buddha, calling him a fool, arrogantly ridiculing him in any way he could.

Finally, after three days of this, the rude traveler couldn't stand it any longer. He asked Buddha, "How can you continue to be so kind and loving when all I've done for the last three days is dishonor, offend and try to find ways to hurt you? Each time I try to hurt you, you respond in a kind manner. How can this be?" Buddha responded with a question for his fellow traveler, "If someone offers you a gift, and you do not accept that gift, to whom the gift belongs?"

—*Zen Tale*

You have the power to accept or reject the circumstances & behaviors. Choose to accept the good and refuse the negative. Return back to the sender, please!

Awareness

"Pain is inevitable. Suffering is optional."

—Haruki Murakami

This is one of the mantras I try to live by whenever things go wrong. We can choose to panic and let our stories spiral out of control or we can take the high road and shift our perspective. I hope you choose the latter. Throughout life we will get all sorts of difficult situations, we always have a choice to react or respond. We can choose to let the pain take over us or rise above it. Make a wise choice because every single choice you make orchestrates your future. Suffering is always a sign that you are not in sync with your real true self. It clearly indicates that you are not in harmony with the vibrations meant for you.

"Anything that annoys you is teaching you patience. Anyone who abandons you is teaching you how to stand up on your own two feet. Anything that angers you is teaching you forgiveness and compassion. Anything that has power over you is teaching you how to take your power back. Anything you hate is teaching you unconditional love. Anything you fear is teaching you courage to overcome your fear. Anything you can't control is teaching you how to let go."

—Jackson Kiddard

It's not you; it's them

This is a very powerful thought. When someone treats you badly, it's truly his or her pain and suffering spilling out on you. Though it's easier said than done, try not to take it personally. Understand where they are; try and see their situation, and if you can help them and you have the strength to, by all means, do. If not, then walk away, because they will keep breaking you down. That's what they feed on. Don't let them.

"There are some people who seem angry and continuously look for conflict; Walk away; the battle they are fighting is not with you, it is with themselves."

—Anonymous

The Decision

December 2013

I filed for Divorce.

"As I walked out the door towards my freedom, I knew that if I did not leave all the anger, hatred, and bitterness behind, I would still be in prison."

—Nelson Mandela

This was the most liberating feeling I had ever experienced. It took a lot of courage, strength, and patience, but it was worth every moment that I experienced after this decision. This was my freedom with myself. I was whole, I wasn't shattered anymore and I had succeeded in getting myself back. I was walking towards the life of my dreams and it felt beautiful. As I was leaving the door of his house, my last words to him were,

"I hope you find the money you've always run after and I hope I find the love I've always dreamt of."

"Never be afraid to fall apart because it is an opportunity to rebuild yourself the way you wish you had been all along."

—Rae Smith

I was 37 years old at that time. I had two beautiful sons and my whole life ahead of me. I was a blank canvas that I could paint however I wished. I converted this painful event in my life to the most positive future. I was no longer a slave to someone else's dream; someone who didn't respect and love me. I was the master of my own life. I made a list of my dreams, my aspirations, and my happiness and then designed my life according to that.

I was content, I had my kids with me, my 'design business' reached a great level of success and I was the highest-paid consultant in my field. I painted regularly and read daily. I was surrounded by beautiful souls. I was also in the best physical state of my life. I took care of myself. Those were basic goals that I had for myself to be achieved within a year and I felt proud in succeeding for my own self.

I managed to get back on my feet very quickly yet there was a deep void inside. This yearning leading to unlimited reading, searching, learning, and thinking, which resulted in the most valuable transformation of my being; the start of my path to Sufism and my spiritual journey.

Lessons, Redirections & Turning Points

Every soul is different and every experience changes you differently. It's mostly how you respond to the experience that makes the difference. Life is a mix of good and bad; an echo of negative and positive. You decide the gift you want to receive and make that happen for you. When something positive comes your way, embrace it, experience it, enjoy it, and be thankful. When something negative comes your way don't panic and retrieve into darkness. Accept, focus, analyze, and learn the lesson it brings you and turn it into an opportunity for growth and betterment.

"When it's time for something new, you will feel it. You will feel a desire to let go, to shed layers, to move, to recreate. You will know because there will be subtle shifts around you. You will release the old because you are really clearing the path for what's ahead. Trust this process. Know that life does not take from us anything unless there is something else imminently awaiting its replacement."

—Brianna West

I learned to honor myself, to prioritize myself, to nurture myself, to constantly learn, create, improve, evolve, live, smile, and respond instead of reacting. I learned through this journey that you should never be dependent on anything or anyone. Work on yourself to be a completely independent soul. Be happy and contented with your life; do what you love; create your own world and once you achieve this, then look for a partner that compliments you and your world.

This is the only earth experience we are getting so let's make the best of it and prioritize our dreams and goals. It's beautiful to give, love, care, and be there for your loved ones but there is a very fine line between being treasured and being taken for granted.

Honor your instincts

Always trust your instincts. Every time you experience a sinking feeling in your gut, identify it, accept & acknowledge. Learn to notice the red flags, learn to trust your inner feelings, learn to trust your instincts, and identify negativity. Every experience is a message, a lesson, a direction, a redirection & it's up to you how to interpret and use this for the best. Major incidents in life are usually redirections & eventually turning points. If you perform an analysis of your past years, you will realize that the negative & positive incidents in your life were major turning points. It's up to you how to use this information, decode & redirect it in your favor and blessings. There is a good in every bad and there is a negative in every positive, we just have to learn to identify and channel it in the correct manner.

Finally, after years, I had a beautiful moment in my life. A Sufi soul, a coworker who I was good friends with proposed to me. That moment came as a huge surprise as he was going through his own healing. It was a beautiful decision and I cherish this soul every day of my life. We sync so effortlessly. We have been married for almost two years now and I pray that whatever time or moments we have together are peaceful, soulful & beautiful. He is such a gentle soul, romantic, spiritual, caring & loving. Thank you, universe!

"And suddenly you know it's time to start something new and trust the magic of new beginnings."

—Eckhart Tolle

We as souls will keep looking for our soulmate until we find them. If we do get attached to a different soul not meant for us through marriage or love, it will eventually end. And when we find our soulmate, the one we are meant to be with, there will not be the temporary excitement but peace in our heart. We will be in the calmest state radiating happiness.

Look around; so many souls are in compromised relationships, trying to make it work. Sad inside; they are at war every single day with themselves. I look at my pictures from my past years and I had lifeless eyes and a sad soul. Today I feel alive because I'm happy. My soul is synced with my purpose, my goals, myself, and who I am meant to be with at this time, in these moments, and for this journey.

"Never be afraid of how deeply or passionately you loved someone who destroyed you, because destroying things is just who they are, but loving deeply and passionately is who you are."

—*Butterflies Rising*

Part 2

Spiritual & Holistic Wellness; The Beginning

A New Chapter In my Life that will change your life

"To begin, begin."

—William Wordsworth

Decades of interest in honoring the earth and trusting in nature to heal, I experienced and learnt tons of information that led me to the path of healing myself, experiencing my own genesis; a re-birth & evolving towards a high vibrational lifestyle. Through many trials and errors, I finally found the purpose of my life; my 'Ikigai'. It has been a very long journey these past years of healing, learning, creating, exploring & finding myself.

"Start by doing what is necessary; then do what's possible and suddenly you are doing the impossible."

—St. Francis of Assisi

I strongly believe that you should find the purpose of your life; Your 'GIFT' and then give it away. Over the years that I dedicated to my own self, I learnt immense amount of valuable information regarding living your life a certain way that heals you, raises your vibration, and syncs you to the earth's energy, hence providing you guidance to where you are meant to be.

It has been a very long journey for the past years of experiencing & healing. I learnt survival, healing, and living all over again. Events & people happen to us and we don't understand why. We resist and hate, we judge and fill ourselves with anger. What we don't realize is that everything is happening for a reason. I'm honored to share all this information with you to help you find your purpose, heal, transform, and live your best life possible.

I started writing this book after the incident that changed my life in 2012. What I experienced after that incident is far more valuable than the suffering the incident caused. The awareness that we have the ability to choose how we respond to an event or experience is our biggest strength. We can't control when something happens to us but we can control our response to it. A negative experience can shatter us completely but our attitude, our choice on how to respond and our power stays with us. When we are at a point in life when everything seems to be finished; the powerful thought & reality is that, the particular moment, in reality, is a new beginning; a rebirth.

We experience the direction of our life's purpose by different sources that nudge us to our purpose. Some of us are very clear on our life paths but many of us are not. I found my life's purpose after rising from an extremely painful experience with faith, courage, and optimism for future. Suffering is always a redirection; if we believe.

The suffering I experienced that made me literally suicidal; also gave me my life's purpose because I chose to rise than lose hope.

My purpose is to be a source to heal your soul and show you the path to genesis, rebirth, and living again. It's not easy but small steps & changes every day will slowly help you rise up from the negative thoughts and environment raising you upwards towards the light and optimism.

"Everything can be taken from a man but one thing; the last of the human freedoms, to choose one's attitude in any given set of circumstances, to choose one's own way."

—Viktor Frankl

When we go through an extremely negative experience our mind, body & soul goes through stages. The painful experience can be anything like loss of a loved one, grief, abuse, financial crisis, family crisis, health crisis, etc. anything that takes away your life and throws you in severe pain is a negative experience for you. The first stage is shock; our mind goes in complete numb mode and halts everything immediately. We don't accept what just happened and we stop feeling, seeing, and experiencing anything else around us. We are stuck in that moment that just altered our life completely. We get in a denial, shock, numbness, and lifeless state. We immediately create an iron wall around us and we guard our aura with everything we can. This is emotional death for us and we feel literally like an emotionless being walking around. There is nothing normal in our state now. We experienced something that changed our life completely and now we don't want to feel anything at all.

"With the end of uncertainty there came the uncertainty

of the end."

—Viktor Frankl

After this stage passes, we enter the bitterness & anger state. We feel bitter about everything around us. Happiness repels us, people who smile irritate our aura. We are in constant fight with ourselves. We are in endless dialogue with our inner state as to why it happened and why us. We feel revengeful and hateful; extremely pessimistic. The agony, the resentment, the injustice, the helplessness, the unreasonableness of it all consumes us completely. This extreme agitation continues and turns into the next state; depression where we stop being bitter and angry and start losing hope for everything. We get into the lowest state of our aura and surround ourselves with negativity and pessimism, sadness, and darkness.

This is the exact state where we can let go and stay this way all our life or surrender to that incident, accept the change that it has brought and rise up from this darkness towards a re-birth, a genesis, a new life filled with acceptance, healing, happiness, positivity, goals, dreams, learning, creativity, evolvement, peace, joy, success, abundance & prosperity.

Every single person who has chosen to let-go of this last state and rise up to a rebirth has found everything they have ever dreamt of as the rising soul from the darkness to light always has more courage, more strength, more faith, more passion, more humbleness, and more will-power; that ultimately sculpts their life exactly how they always wanted and I say this from personal experience. We can't control what happens to us but we can control how we respond to it. We can let the incident define and direct our life or we rise up from this and we can define and direct our life ourselves.

We can let this negative overpower our entire being or we can take the reins back in our hands and turn this negative into the biggest positive for us. We

can't undo what happened but we can outdo our current state and choose to live the best life possible.

The universe is constantly responding to our thoughts. So, whatever we are experiencing at that particular moment is the universe synchronizing events to give us exactly what we are asking. If we stay in negativity, we will attract the exact frequency and when we start letting go and raising our vibrations the universe will start aligning us to experiences of the new vibration.

All that happened in my life was a massive learning experience and redirection towards my purpose. Suffering is painful, but we can choose to rise above it slowly with a guideline to come out of it eventually following the steps narrated in the following chapters. The steps written are a synopsis of everything that helped me heal and rise above my situation. It took me many years of learning, reading, analyzing, experiencing, and eventually applications of it all.

It took me many years to mentally let-go of that exact moment in my life when my ex-husband hit me. The look in his eyes and the helplessness in my being, the beast in him and the hurt in me, the condescending act and my soul under attack, the strength of his hand and the sharp pain I felt, the evil in his eyes and the shock in my soul, the power play on his side and the moment of weakness within me. Those moments made me feel like a worthless creature in a wild unjust world being treated in the most demeaning manner, in the most spur of the moment attack by an evil entity who was far more physically strong and making use of that strength at the time to cause pain to someone far weaker than him in strength, caught off guard completely and in a state of utter shock. My body was bruised so badly that I could not even walk, I fell down and passed out waking up to the first state; utter shock.

Pain is pain, suffering is suffering & hurt is hurt. There is no level or state from low to high. When you are in pain there is no rating of that pain. We can't judge if someone is in more pain or less depending on their suffering. But now when I look back after letting-go of this moment from my mind, body & soul, I feel that every moment of my life makes sense now.

If we choose to rise above our suffering, we grow beyond our limits emotionally, spiritually & mentally. We have the choice to turn our life around to the greatest possible life from this moment onwards or to choose to let-go, suffer & vegetate our mind, body & soul ultimately decaying to death.

We can choose every day of our life to be the best day possible or we can let all negativity consume our thoughts and direct our day & life accordingly.

This world is full of good & bad, evils & saints, negative & positive. You can choose to attract everything positive, and you can, with faith but you should also be prepared to handle the negative if it comes. There is an evil in every corner of your life and there is a saint as well. You get to experience it all and the power of your attitude and response carves out your life accordingly.

I was always meant to help, to heal, to be a medium for souls who are hurting helping them to rise above their pain. Helping souls who are hurting or living with a void to find their purpose & meaning. Fast forward all these years and I am on my 'Sufi' and 'Spiritual' journey, a holistic & high vibrational lifestyle practitioner, my sons are grown up and they are the best part of my life, I'm writing, traveling to experience beautiful countries and cultures, conducting 'Healing Hour/ Zikr' and I have a beautiful loving partner right next to me in my journey. My life revolves around what I thought could never happen and it started with the choice I made to heal, encompassed by very strong faith & commitment.

"Those who know how close the connection is between the state of mind of a man- his courage and hope, or lack of them – and the state of immunity of his body will understand that the sudden loss of hope and courage can have a deadly effect."

—*Viktor Frankl*

High Vibrational Lifestyle

"If you want to find the secrets of the universe, think in terms of Energy, Frequency & Vibration."

—Nikola Tesla

We identify ourselves as physical entities but in reality, we are spiritual beings having a human experience in a physical body. We are 'Energy', 'Frequency', and 'Vibration'. Our existence is vibrational. Every cell in our body is in momentum; this is our reality.

Vibration is the frequency of our mind, body, and soul. It's the energy that encompasses our being. It is a direct result of how we have lived your life so far, every thought that has ever generated in our mind, every experience that we have ever had, and every moment that we have taken breath has resulted in the frequency that we are at right now. Our vibration is our legend; our personal definition. It's our essence and our gift. There is no one else like us in this entire universe. We are unique and special in your own vibrational manner. Our current vibration is in direct proportion to our thoughts, beliefs, spoken words, our behavior, attitude, perceptions, persona, aura, actions and reactions.

The higher our vibration, the lighter we hold and there is sacred poetic flow of energy inside and outside us. The higher our vibration is; the stronger we are connected to our source. Our eternal source energy; our legend. High vibration feelings are love, happiness, compassion, kindness, serenity, peace, warmth, calmness, forgiveness, awareness, joy and contentment etc.

If our vibration is low then our entire being is in a state of negativity and hardship. Our energy will be heavy and stagnant. Our mind body and soul will not be aligned and in flow. Low Vibration feelings are fear, sadness, anger, resentment, guilt, blame, judgement, shame, addictions, greed and jealousy etc. We have the absolute potential to raise our vibration as high as we desire. In other words, this is the path to enlightenment and a return to one's true spiritual legend.

When we want something in our life, we have to understand its frequency, to change and alter our life and body's frequency to match the frequency of our dream. That's how we achieve our dreams and what we desire. We learn what frequency it's at and we raise our frequency to match that particular frequency, hence resulting in achievement. Some call it the 'Law of attraction'. I call it learning the 'art of energy'. Every Living thing is made up of energy and energy is vibrating at a certain frequency, our task is to match the frequency of what we desire. Yes, it is that simple!

This is harmony, being aligned to our source, our purpose, our mantra, our dreams, and our goals. It's our 'FLOW', our 'ALIGNMENT'. In the older times there was one TV channel and we had to 'TUNE' to a certain number to watch. This concept is exactly that 'Tuning Code'. If we stop at the wrong code the channel will not come on, in fact we will hear the buzzing static noises. Our goal is to find that perfect code and tune our life to that frequency in order to achieve that goal or dream.

Match the frequency of what you want. For that you have to practice the art of concentration. Concentrate on the particular GOAL or DREAM, visualize it every single day with strong emotions, feel yourself experiencing it and it will eventually manifest. Yes, it will!

We are energetic beings in physical bodies. Our thoughts are extremely powerful. If we realize the power of our thoughts in shaping our life and your destiny, we will not let a single negative thought appear or stay in our brain. We need to be very mindful of what we think. We become what we think and ultimately what we say.

Diligently become aware of what you think and say as this becomes your reality.

All souls vibrate energetically at a particular frequency. You either vibrate at the lower end of the frequency level or higher. High vibrations are associated with positive qualities and feelings, such as love, forgiveness, compassion, and peace. On the other hand, low vibrations are associated with qualities such as hatred, fear, greed, and depression.

The higher the frequency of your energy or vibration, the lighter you feel in your physical and mental realm. Your mind, body, and soul energy will be full of (Nur) light! You feel in control of your life and experience greater personal power, clarity, love, serenity, and happiness. You may have very less or no pain in your physical body. You feel more in grasp of your emotions. Your life attracts what is best for you and your purpose. Everything flows with synchronicity, and you manifest what you desire with ease. Your life has a beautiful strong positive aura.

As you elevate to a higher level of consciousness and vibration your awareness, thoughts, words, and consciousness ascend accordingly and strengthen you immensely.

The lower the frequency, the heavier your energy, and more difficult your problems seem. You experience pain and discomfort in your physical body, strong negative emotions and mental confusion. Mentally you don't feel clarity for anything and physically your energy feels darker. You feel lethargic with a negative aura around you. Despair, sadness, depression, anxiety will consume you if you are vibrating at a lower frequency. You don't feel in control of anything around yourself. There is strongly a negative aura.

Have you ever felt that when you are around certain kind of souls, your energy just naturally rises, you feel synced in, and you feel full of life and happy? Those are high frequency souls and you are drawn to them like a strong magnet. Their aura attracts you. Their presence makes you relaxed and you feel full of life.

Now notice the souls that drain your energy, the toxic aura souls. They are the ones you need to stay distant from. They suck the happiness out of your system and before you know it you are out of sync, restless, and maybe even in anxiety. Living your life in a higher vibration state is going to become more and more vital to you as you learn more about it and realize how everything in your life changes for the best once you start raising your vibrations. Choosing the light of a higher vibration requires a firm commitment and follow through plan in your daily life.

"We are not wanting you to seek control over your environment at all. We want you to seek control over your vibration and Law of Attraction will take care of the Environment."

—Abraham-Hicks

We are meant to have fun and enjoy being on 'Earth'. Life is not a punishment; in fact, it's an opportunity to learn lessons through experiences and rise. It's a journey where we are meant to feel real joy and happiness. It's not what happens to us that matters so much, it is our attitude and response to what happens that matters. We are a tiny speck of sand in the ocean of life. Live your life to its fullest. Focus on your journey and not the result. Let go of all regrets and the past. Live a life filled with love for your 'Universal Power', yourself, and everyone on this and other planets. I love the following prayer that helps me put many issues into a healthier and more balanced perspective.

"God grant me the serenity to accept the things I cannot change, courage to change the things I can, and wisdom to know the difference."

—Anonymous

Making a commitment to live a high vibrational lifestyle requires a firm plan and very strong willpower. It all comes down to what is the priority in your life. Do you want to keep living the way you are living right now? Ask yourself these questions at this moment:

- Are you happy where you are in life right now?
- Are you happy with the person you have become?
- Are you happy with your emotional & physical state?

If the answer is YES, then congratulations, you are experiencing a high vibrational state. Please keep doing whatever you are practicing and keep going higher. If you answered NO, then you have two choices:

- Either you can do nothing and stay in this state; which will surely keep getting worse hence resulting in a downward spiral of low vibrational life ahead.
- OR you can COMMIT to yourself, take a firm decision and RISE up from all this to a better state and ultimately a beautiful high vibrational life; which is what I chose.

"The person you'll be in five years depends largely on the information you feed your mind today. Be picky about the books you read, the people you spend time with, and the conversations you engage in."

—Ruben Chavez

By becoming the best version of yourself, you can also help others do the same, and ultimately lead humanity to a more positive high frequency state. Whatever you do in life, never retire. Keep adding purpose to your life and life will keep becoming more beautiful. Take care of your health by incorporating the 7 zones in your day and you will always be in optimum health & alignment.

"When you want something, all the universe conspires in helping you to achieve it."

—Paulo Coelho

You are constantly creating who you are

- What you eat becomes your body
- What you feel becomes your mood
- What you think becomes your mind
- What you love becomes your passion
- What you say becomes your reality
- What you see becomes your perspective
- What you connect to becomes your spirit
- What you allow becomes your destiny

Everything in life is things you've attracted. Take responsibility of it all. You are not attracting the negative things consciously but subconsciously you may not even know what you are constantly thinking about. We attract what we think about. Consciously change your thoughts to positive & happy ones. Then you'll see things changing. Imagine a lit ball of Light (Nur). Imagine all your dreams there and forget about the black ball of negativity or sadness.

"Whether you think you can or whether you think you can't. You're right either way."

—Henry Ford

Instead of searching for the endless treasure, gift the world; the best service that you're capable of. Count your blessings if you want to stop worrying and start living. Count your blessings and not your troubles.

"I had the blues because I had no shoes...until upon the street I met a man who had no feet."

—Denis Waitley

Emotional Energy Evolution (EEE)

Emotions are our body's way of expressing its current state and vibrational level. Our body is the most magnificent entity which gives signals itself to let us know what needs to be taken care of; only if we understand this mechanism and pay attention to the signals, mainly our 'EEE' state.

Awareness is the key to understanding where you are and where you need to be. A deep analysis of your emotional state can identify the level that you are at and the steps you need to take to take care of it. The EEE (Emotional Energy Evolution) chart below is a guide for you to understand which phase, stage, and level you currently are. Once you understand your current level of 'Emotional Energy' state, you will have the awareness to improve your vibrational state to bring yourself to the desired 'EEE-Level'.

EEE – Level 1	EEE- Level 2	EEE- Level 3	EEE-Level 4
Ecstasy	Insecurity	Ego battles	
Passion	Pessimism	Bitterness	Evilness
Happiness	Overwhelm-ness	Hatred	
Optimism	Fear	Anger	
Positivity	Doubt	Revenge	
Contentment	Frustration	Jealousy	
Freedom	Blame	Competition	
Happiness	Discouragement		
Love	Impatience		
Lightness in being	Constant worry		
Tranquility	Sadness		

What is your EEE Level? The following chapters will give you awareness & guide you in detail how to improve your EEE level and raise your vibrations.

Purpose of Life & its Vitality

You have the freedom to pursue your own unique path and it is up to you to reclaim your divine magic to create the life you want.

I have spent almost 43 years on this beautiful earth and finally in my 40th year of life I started realizing what my purpose was. 40 is a beautiful age I must say. I would say 40 is the age where your naive years actually and officially end. You finally start getting an idea about life.

The journey to realizing and finding my own purpose was quite a ride & collection of experiences. I was always the wild child looking for the spiritual essence of life. People & places were all part of the 'Earth' experience for me and my thirst of traveling and getting to know people and different cultures only became stronger with age. As a teenager from the eastern culture, having a Master's degree is a necessity not a choice. I did my Masters in Mass Communication and eventually started my 'Interior Design' business as a complete change of career when we moved back. I had decorated my own home and started getting inquiries about design. Having no 'Design Degree', I started refusing until one day I thought this may be it. To me this became my calling or at least I thought. I did every course that I could to learn design professionally and lead a high achieving design firm for almost a decade.

My first project of Interior design was a 12,000 sq. ft. home in DHA, Lahore. I accepted the project and the clients were extremely happy with the results. This was another life-changing moment for me as I became the highest-paid interior designer at that moment in my first project. I thanked God for that achievement and started working dedicatedly in the design industry working on over 200 projects within the next few years. I was financially stable and thought this was what I was always meant to do.

At the peak of my career, the unthinkable in my personal life happened that shook me to my core. The incident that changed everything in my life.

"Sometimes the bad things that happen in our lives put us directly on the path to the best things that will ever happen to us."

—Nicole Reed

Fast forward 7 years and here I am writing this book. At this point in my life, I have so much clarity as to why everything happened. It all had a purpose. The purpose was to jolt me out of a negative situation and redirect me to my path & calling. Now that I think about it there were many moments when the universe was giving me signs to leave the toxic environment but I wasn't ready to leave. I was trying to "Band-Aid" the situation and carry on with my life. We all do this many times in our lives when we are trying to make it work but the effort is worthless as the universe wants us to take the courage and leap of faith and remove ourselves from the situation.

The years of my life after that incident were a journey of healing and finding myself, journey of self-awareness, journey of learning, and identifying my purpose. I went through extreme phases of loneliness, depression, serenity, calmness, spiritual growth & learning, eventually bringing me to where I am today. I used to crave for the experience of "happiness" and "being aligned to my purpose & source". I had no idea how! I used to wake up every day with the thirst to find out but had no direction.

I used to see 'happy' people and those moments were so intense for me as I didn't know how to be happy. I used to keep recalling the last time in my life that I felt aligned and the memories from two decades back used to appear. I craved the feeling of 'being home'. Something was missing in my life before; a huge void. I used to brush it off thinking its depression or I'm not grateful as I was living a good life financially. My personal life was on the rocks and my mental health was in extreme low vibration because of it. But one thing that I used to do as a hobby always sparked a light in me and I used to get a high out of it. It was talking to friends or loved ones in need and helping them get through their problems. The feeling of helping and healing someone and raising the vibration to their best self through therapy, positivity, healing words, guidance, nutrition & rituals, gave me ultimate happiness. I couldn't do a lot of it as my own energy was at a low state most of the times. But any chance that I got I loved healing souls.

One day I carved out a formal therapy plan and started doing this professionally on the side helping people with therapy sessions and leaving those sessions with the ultimate feeling of accomplishment and raised vibration. Over time those people healed and got back in their lives with the utmost high state of vibration achieving their goals and dreams. Their messages of gratitude were my therapy and my addiction. Nothing made me feel more empowered and fulfilled than knowing that I made a difference in someone's life and helped them achieve their goals.

At the same time, I was extremely busy with my design business and everything that was happening in my personal life. What I didn't realize at that time was that healing and helping people was my purpose in life, as it gave me the strength and happiness that I was craving. We all think that if we are making money then this is the right path. The right path is actually when we are in complete alignment with ourselves and our purpose; that's when we feel fulfilled.

I was always inspired by my grandmother's beliefs and faith in' Mother Earth's' healing powers. She used to believe strongly in healing through nutrition and nature's power and its extreme benefits to the human body. As a young girl I used cook and decorate my plate like art. I used to always make own skincare. I used to be in my mother's kitchen making my own scrubs and masks. To this day I make and use my own skincare and believe strongly in honoring the 'Earth' and having faith in its healing and nourishing powers. I'm extremely fascinated by the treasure that mother earth has given us in forms of plants and their healing properties. Fruits, vegetables, nuts, and seeds inspire me every single day for healing, nourishing, skincare, and raising one's vibrations.

Today as I am writing this book it makes me smile that I thought design was my purpose and I didn't realize for decades that almost everything that I was doing in my entire day besides design, was my purpose. Yes, it took me years and years to find that out and that's the reason why I am writing this book which I started. I'm writing to help and heal you. I'm writing this book to make you aware and to help you raise your vibrations so you can achieve everything that you have always wanted. I'm writing this to help you align to your source and purpose.

How did I figure out my purpose? Over years and years, I asked myself these questions:

- What makes me happy?
- What am I here to do?
- What's my purpose on this earth?

- Why do I feel depressed?
- Why is there a void in my heart?
- Why do I not feel fulfilled?
- What is missing?
- Why me?
- What is wrong with me?

Eventually, I realized that I was asking myself the wrong questions. The right questions can't be vague and negative. The right questions started appearing when I surrendered to the universe (God) finally. I surrendered to the flow and asked for help and guidance. Then I finally started realizing the right questions:

- What sparks a light in me?
- What makes me forget the whole world around me?
- What is my skill and talent?
- What was I passionate about as a child?
- If I had no financial responsibilities, how would I spend my day?
- What do I wait for with passion and drive?
- What is the one thing I do that makes time fly?
- What conversations do I love having with my friends and loved ones?
- What is in my bucket list?
- What are the moments that I feel happiest, what am I doing at that time, who am I with, what am I talking about?
- When was the last moment I felt on top of this world? What was I doing?

- How do I want people to remember me when I leave this earth?
- What do I love searching about?
- Looking at my books, what do I love reading about?
- Looking at my weekends, what activities do I wait to get to?
- What makes me unique from others?
- What I may take as my weakness, could be my biggest strength, what is my weakness?
- What is my strength?
- How would a friend define me today?
- What do I think I waste time on?
- What is my "I wish.... statement?" What do I wish for?
- If I knew today that I only had one year to live, what will I do, how will I live the next 365 days?
- What do I do when I am stressed?
- How do I relieve my stress?
- Where does my mind wander when I am sitting by myself?
- What are the moments in life that I have experienced a sudden surge of energy and passion run through me and my heart immediately says, I want this experience in my life?

No question is wrong and no answer is weird. Go through these questions every day for 7 days and write answers to each and in 7 days you will find your reason for existence, your purpose, your direction. It maybe vague but when you re-read your answers you will find clues to the direction of your life and what you are meant to do. Repeat this exercise every year to refresh your path and mind.

Sometimes a certain portion of our life is dedicated to a certain purpose and once it's fulfilled, you move on to a different or higher purpose in the same realm.

I found my purpose at this stage of my life by going through these questions numerous times and analyzing answers over and over again. Another exercise is to ask a few of your closest loved ones to send you a few lines describing you. What do they think your strengths and weaknesses are? This was also a great eye-opener. Sometimes we think of us in a different way compared to who we actually are. We are extremely critical of our own self and sometimes we don't even realize what our skills and talents are. This exercise of asking loved ones is a great way to look at yourself through the eyes of different souls.

It took many years and many painful and happy moments but I achieved what I was looking for. The void in me filled with the energy of knowing my purpose. I finally had a direction and that's the most beautiful and contended feeling anyone can experience.

My purpose in life at this stage of my existence is to raise the vibrations of souls in need, help them align to their source and being. Heal them find their purpose, their ikigai, and help them align their life the right way for them. Help them heal their pain and direct them to their purpose. With that my passion is honoring the 'Earth' and utilizing the treasures given to us by nourishing our mind, body & soul via living a high vibrational lifestyle through rituals & nutrition.

This year I have committed myself to finish writing this book that I started in year 2012. This book to become a massive healing source to all souls by healing their pain, helping them align their life and to help them find their purpose.

A few weeks back I wrote my mission statement and it is;

"Helping souls achieve a high vibrational lifestyle through rituals, nutrition, and my writings. Honoring the earth and its intricate cycles of life and using the valuable information to help souls achieve wellness."

When you find your purpose write your mission statement. All it encompasses is what your heart desires. Reading it every day will give you guidance and direction

Your purpose

The purpose for all of us who come to this world is to constantly advance and expand our collective consciousness, align ourselves with the universe, and flow. We are all on this earth with a purpose; every single one of us. The idea is to find our particular purpose to help humanity to its utmost level. The way our inner self is looking for our purpose is the same manner in which our purpose is trying to find its way to us as it's linked to us by the universe. When we discover our purpose, it will take away this void that we have deep in our heart and soul giving us the ultimate feeling of contentment. Our entire life will start making sense and we will understand the deeper meaning behind everything that has happened in our life so far on our journey.

"What you seek is seeking you."

—Rumi

The void, the emptiness, the meaninglessness, the feeling of not knowing what to do with our life goes away once we have our purpose in front of us. Any suffering that we are rising from will have a deeper meaning when all the pain is channeled towards achieving our purpose.

"He who has a 'why' to live for can bear almost any 'how'."

—Friedrich Nietzsche

Life becomes so contented and meaningful when we find our true calling; our purpose. It's the beautiful unique trait we have that empowers our soul and brings happiness & benefit to others. And yes, it's an entire process that we go through just to find our calling, our purpose. When we finally find our calling, we will see traces of it over the last decades of our life. We will notice the pattern and the path that lead to where we are at that moment. Everything happens for a reason. Every event and person has a purpose and we will understand this once we reach and identify our calling. That's the moment that will change us inside out. When we will stop blaming others and understand why everything in our life happened. When we immerse ourselves in our calling, this is the highest vibration that we can ever be in. It's Enchanting!

When you start raising your vibration intentionally, magic starts to happen in your life. You attract high vibrational people and events and soon you are only surrounded by the best energy and frequency, hence enhancing your life immensely. Surrendering to your present is the first step; don't resist anything. Just accept your life first as is and then slowly and intentionally follow the guidelines in this book and watch your life change and your purpose being exposed to you with utmost clarity & direction.

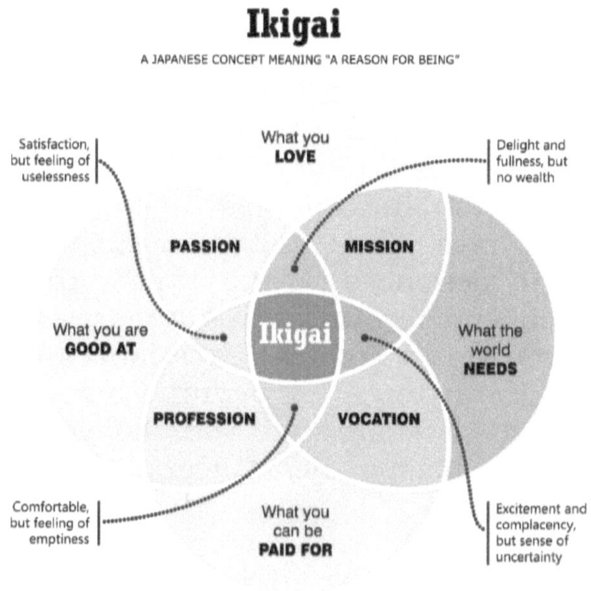

Ikigai

A JAPANESE CONCEPT MEANING "A REASON FOR BEING"

Satisfaction, but feeling of uselessness

What you LOVE

Delight and fullness, but no wealth

PASSION

MISSION

What you are GOOD AT

Ikigai

What the world NEEDS

PROFESSION

VOCATION

Comfortable, but feeling of emptiness

What you can be PAID FOR

Excitement and complacency, but sense of uncertainty

In Japanese, Ikigai is written in a way that it means "Life to be worthwhile". What makes us enjoy doing something so much that we forget about any stress or worries and 'BE' in that moment. Anything that gives us the 'POWER' of 'BEING IN THE NOW' is our purpose. When we are completely immersed in the activity that we forget the existence of the world; that's our ikigai, our purpose. We need to focus on all the activities that bring us in this state of flow, the state of being, and the state of now. This is the state when we are aligned with the vibrations of the universe connected to our purpose.

Energy, Frequency, Vibration & Emotions

There is a magnificent source of energy inside you. It is not the energy that you get from your daily nourishment, rest, or from any outer source. This energy originates from your divine infinite source and is endless. You are powerful beyond your own thoughts. This powerful energy is strong, abundant & endless. If you don't feel it then you have blocked it with holding on to negative experiences. Untie those knots, free your soul, and tap into this ultimate reserve of energy to magnify your life experiences. You can tap into it anytime you want. This energy is stored in the 7 chakras of your body. The root, sacral, solar plexus, heart, throat, third eye & crown chakra.

Achieve the state of peace, love, tranquility, contentment, serenity, happiness & joy by unblocking all your chakras, untying all the knots in your soul that are blocked energies. Open your heart, be receptive, allow experiences to flow through you, and not stay causing energy stagnancy.

In the Gospel of Thomas found in Egypt, it says "Ask Without hidden motives and be surrounded by your answer. Be Enveloped by what you desire, that your gladness be full."

A very important aspect I learnt was not to resist, judge, or blame a situation. For e.g. in china practitioners healed cancer tumor from a woman with chanting, faith, belief, and meditation. How? They didn't blame, reject, or judge cancer. They accepted it as a possibility and then intended for a new reality. They accepted the tumor as in the quantum world anything is possible. They didn't hate cancer; they didn't resent it. They didn't curse it instead they accepted the situation first as is without any judgment or threat. And then intended for a new reality by feeling emotionally, physically, and mentally that the woman is healed. They chanted the words 'healing' and 'now' to make it a reality in that moment of time without any ego, resentment, negativity, fear, or judgment to cancer, they accepted its presence and released the emotion for a new reality.

In the quantum world physical reality responds to the language of the universe and the language of the universe is 'energy' which initiates from thoughts, feelings & emotions. The power of your mind is beyond measure. The power of your feelings is beyond infinite. You create your reality by how you feel, what you say, and what you think.

Learn to Flow

Learn to Allow

Learn to Receive

Learn to be Happy

Learn to Float with the energy of the universe

Learn to let go

Learn to Breathe without guilt or fear

Learn to Inhale & exhale without pressure

Learn to live without feeling overwhelmed

You are here on this earth to be happy and joyous. The universe wants you to enjoy this experience. There is enough in this universe for every single one of us. We don't owe anyone anything and if we ask for ourselves, we don't deprive anyone of anything. When we are healthy and well, we don't say to ourselves that this is enough now it's someone else's turn to be healthy. We enjoy that state forever. And in the same manner, there is enough abundance for everyone in their vortex in this quantum zone. You just have to tap in and receive.

Align with your energy source in such a way that there is no resistance, so it flows effortlessly in your life. In the quantum world of energy & vibration, there is no resistance or effort. These are only present outside the zone. Once you align yourself with the zone there is no need for any effort, resistance, or fear. 'FLOW' is the key, learn to swim with the current without any effort of changing anything yourself. Allow your source to make the changes and it will turn your flow smoothly towards your destiny without any jolts or resistance. You will flow like water towards the life you belong to.

You can't orchestrate your destiny through physical action, you can sit back, relax, and allow the universe to orchestrate the energy towards you and your dreams. The high vibrational energy vibrates where it is intended and allowed without resistance, fear, judgment, or ego.

You are here on this earth to be happy. There is no pain, it's all illusion. Detachment is the key to a happy fulfilled life. Don't get attached to anything or anyone in this world. Be attached to your source. It's who you are and where you belong. Everything else and everyone else around you are the other players in the game of earth. They will come and go as per their vibrational vortex. And their presence will alter as per your vibrational level. The ones you lose don't sync with you anymore or their time in your journey is finished. Don't cry over the ones who are no longer on your path. They are not meant to go where you are going and vice versa. Be happy how far you have come along and be extremely excited at where you are headed.

Be in the extreme state of allowing and receiving. Be in a supreme state of high vibrational energy so you attract all that you desire. To be in that state you have to focus and feel. Focus on how you feel and feel the best. Make peace with the authenticity of where you are at this moment of your life. Look back for a moment, the things you overcame, the events you experienced, the people you loved and lost, the life you have lived so far, every single moment, event, experience, and person has shaped you and directed you to where you are today. Nothing was a coincidence. It was all orchestrated by the universe responding to your vibrations.

Take this moment to let go of any pain, hurt, grudge, or hate that you have kept inside for anyone. Accept their role in your life path, acknowledge the lesson learnt, and let them go. Free your soul of their energy and create space for new positive experiences. Close your eyes and connect with the spirit soul of that person one by one and acknowledge them, thank them for their role, forgive them and let them go. Free their spirit energy from your spirit energy, so you create new sacred fresh space for new and better experiences. Clear the clutter from your soul of pain, grief, past, negativity, and hurt. Create space for love, happiness, serenity, dreams, and peace.

The Universe will respond to every single vibration that you are emitting. Be mindful.

Heal Your Heart & Soul

"Ultimately, Healing must be concerned with the evolution of the individual rather than solely with his or her survival."

—Lonny Jarrett

When we view our lives from a sacred higher perspective and vibrational level, we come to terms with the fact that all crisis, trials, negativities, and problems are in fact opportunities for personal and spiritual growth. It is entirely up to us how to depict their reason and learn from them by altering our actions, reactions & responses accordingly.

We need to completely accept our responsibility for our entire life, understanding the fact that we are co-creators of our life experiences. We have to accept that we are not powerless victims of the orchestrated events happening in our lives. The stagnant energy from pain and these traumatic events create negative blocks in our frequency which we need to let go and create space for positive experiences in our lives. When we hold onto negative emotions, we literally store chunks of negative energy from all those people, events, and experiences in our 'Energy Fields', hence limiting ourselves to new positive scared experiences. When we keep ourselves in the place of negativity, judgment, or pain, we lower our vibrations.

In order for us to fully step into our light, resolve our soul's energy, detangle our purpose and raise our vibrations, we must step up, face directly, and clear all those things we refuse to acknowledge from deep inside ourselves. Raising our vibrations and merging with our sacred source requires for us to bring everything we have been avoiding into our conscious awareness so it can be surfaced and healed. This ritual will convert the dark side of our deep soul into light. Energy is always radiating healing energy and it is the best thing to transform the dark energy to light hence attracting and creating space for more goodness in our lives. When we choose to respond positively to a negative event we raise your vibration & activate healing right away. When we forgive the people who hurt us, we immediately raise our frequency.

Pessimism, Rage, Revenge, Anger, Blame, Jealousy, Irritation, Hopelessness, Sadness, Anxiety, Depression, Low Energy, etc. are all indications that we are not in sync with our real self; our sacred source. These are powerful indicators to initiate the healing process in our life. Release all these feelings from your aura & Raise your vibration to initiate the healing process.

Learn to fall in love with yourself first. You are a beautiful, magnificent, and divine being. You are a part of the source energy, you are not separate. No matter what you have experienced or done in your life, your true self, your spirit, your soul remains in a state of perfection. Do not judge yourself ever. Be aware of your actions and if they are low vibrational actions, then correct yourself immediately and aim for better. Forgive yourself first and choose better from this point onwards.

Self-love is extremely vital to our path forward to enlightenment. We need to love and accept every aspect of our beings. We should never compromise the integrity of our souls. We need to choose to be self –fulfilling and stop expecting someone else to provide the love we seek. Unconditional love can only be found within ourselves and our source. Activate your own love, feel it, and be it. Release everything that does not serve you or your highest purpose. Allow yourself to activate the deep intense soul fulfilling love that is in your own soul. You are who you have been waiting for; it is your own love that you seek. When you begin to truly love yourself and remember how extraordinary you truly are, you will connect and merge into the divine sacred source's love. This is beyond human love and is intensely fulfilling. In this state you will attract what is best for your soul; hence the ultimate.

Forgiveness

Forgiving is one of the most powerful ways to raise your vibration because there is nothing holding you down anymore, allowing you to release negative frequencies that you were holding onto. Forgiveness brings peace and harmony to your own soul. It provides you with inner tranquility and the freedom to move on. Once you release that energy from your soul, there is less burden on it to take. Forgiveness is a process of deeply understanding who we are, analyzing our actions and reactions, releasing the pain and hurt and lastly promising ourselves not to put our mind body and soul through another experience like that by intentionally vibrating so high that any low vibrational person, incident or event can ever harm us.

"I asked God why you are taking me through troubled waters. He replied because your enemies can't swim."

—Anonymous

When you don't forgive you are attached to that event or person's spirit energy, which constantly brings your energy down; hence there is a constant connection. Change your perspective and your life will change for the better. Look at someone who has hurt you and focus on that person and experience as your greatest teacher instead of that person as an enemy. Thank their spirit energy to bring you to this incredible moment of clarity, assurance & personal transformation.

"The world isn't filled with haters and toxic people. It is filled with people who are hurting and trying ineffectively, to give themselves relief, so distance yourself if you must, but try to do with empathy, not judgment. The only cure for haters is love, so try to show them more kindness then they showed you. This is how we can slowly make the world a more loving place."

—Lori Deschene

A beautiful Ritual of Forgiveness

- Forgiveness is necessary to release unwanted stagnant energy and create beautiful space for new experiences. Sit in a relaxed beautiful space preferably outside if you can. Think of all the people you have hurt in your life intentionally or unintentionally. One by one speak to each person's spirit energy, acknowledging their part in your life, thank their presence, and ask for forgiveness from the depths of your heart and soul. Sincerely apologize if you have hurt them. Then request that person's spirit energy to release you and your spirit from any energy link whatsoever and release them from your being. Take this moment to make a promise to yourself to never repeat that specific behavior again in your life.

- The second part of this ritual is more beautiful. Think of all the people in your life who have intentionally or unintentionally hurt you. One by one speak to each person's spirit energy, acknowledging their part in your life, letting them know exactly how you feel, thank their presence, and the experience that they offered without judgment. Then from the core of your heart and soul forgive them sincerely then release that person's spirit energy from your heart, soul, mind, and spirit; hence creating a beautiful sacred space for positive experiences to initiate in your life.

This ritual will be life changing for your mind, body and soul. Clearing stagnant painful energy has immense benefits for one's life to continue in its poetic manner

Take Responsibility

If your life is not exactly where you want it to be, take 100% responsibility of it right now. Own your present life and only then can you start to improve from that point onwards. If you waste your day & time complaining and blaming others constantly, you will stay in this low vibrational victim mindset with zero growth. But if you are in desire of a positive life and unlimited success, then choose to be in an "achiever mindset" and get busy creating the life you want instead of complaining. Become so busy creating your positive life that you have absolutely no time to complain. The moment you take 100% responsibility of everything that has happened in your life is the exact miraculous moment you claim your power back and you can achieve anything you ever imagined in your life.

Taking responsibility does not by any means make you take the blame of whatever happened in your life. You are not blaming yourself, you are only taking responsibility of your low vibrational mindset of fear, sadness, negativity, jealousy, your choices, etc. that attracted any negative event in your life and you will change from this moment onwards. Blame targets the reason why the event happened and you are not doing that, you are not blaming yourself. You are taking responsibility and when you do that you transient into the mindset of improving your situation in future.

Step up for your growth, accept 100% responsibility for improving your life and future events.

Take ownership of your life. Don't let external forces direct the course of your life, events, and decisions. When you take responsibility, you rise above the blame game and take charge of your life direction. From here onwards improve your aura, your day and your life will start taking a magnificent course. Analyze and learn from everything that happened. There is a lesson in all events. Extract the essence of your lesson and store it in your mind to be applied in all future endeavors to make sure you don't have to re-live any past experiences. Once you sync into this mindset you are in 100% control of the direction of your life instead of external forces.

"You can't undo the past, but you can sure as hell outdo it."

—Anonymous

Love yourself

"It's time to unlearn the things you learned from wounded people."

—Anonymous

Learn to love yourself; accept your worst self just as you accept your best self. You, yourself are your own best friend, because the only thing that you have control over, in the end, is yourselves. You are extremely valuable, Always make yourself a priority. Respect your boundaries and pay attention to your body, heart, and soul. Incorporate the 7 Zones in your life to raise your vibrations. When you love yourself, forgive yourself and completely accept yourself, you begin to love and accept others as they are as well. This is a great journey that helps you to let go of negative energies & emotions.

When there is no enemy within, the enemy outside can do you no harm."

—African proverb

Awareness of your environment

Analyze your surroundings for toxic people & toxic environment. Be extremely selective and conscious of people you are spending your time with and let go of those who do not serve you now. Your present & your future is on a different path now. Your journey is in ascension and you can't afford to be surrounded by anything that brings you down. Awareness is the first step; as you become aware of your surroundings, their energies & their impact on you, you have the power to change them. This action will start altering your reality and raise your vibration. Your surroundings execute your response & behavior. When you improve your environment; you improve your behavior as a default setting. Doing this ritual with awareness will help you to release the lower vibrations and negative emotions, resulting in raising your vibration and helping you become better.

"Not all toxic people are cruel and uncaring. Some of them love us dearly. Most of them may have good intentions. Most are toxic to our being simply because their needs and way of existing in this world forces us to compromise ourselves and our happiness. They aren't inherently bad people; they just aren't the right people for us. And as

hard as it is, we have to let them go. You have to make your wellbeing a priority. Whether that means breaking up with someone you care about, loving a family member from a distance, letting go of a friend, or removing yourself from a situation that feels painful – you have every right to leave and create a safer space for yourself."

—Daniell Koepke

Let go

"Letting go" is a conscious choice that you make with yourself to elevate from the particular scenario and completely release your mind, body, and soul from it. It's a ritual to release worry, doubt, negativity & fear about the particular situation, person, or the outcome. Letting go is a conscious decision that strengthens your inner being and helps you focus on what you can control instead of being constantly worried about what you can't control. This ritual releases any negative energy that blocks your happiness and no longer serves you on your future journey. Releasing and "Letting Go" removes worry and stagnant energy blocks & enables the doors of brand-new opportunities.

"There is an indescribable peace that settles into your soul space once you lean into the open arms of the universe and surrender. Nothing creates more anxiety than your own expectations of where you believe your life should be. Embrace

where you are. Every chapter has its purpose; it may not seem like it in the moment, but in time, certain lessons will reveal themselves to you. Trust in the magic of divine timings and know that everything that you are asking for, is making its way to you at this very moment. Eliminate the negativity in your mind to make room for the blessings that were carefully tailored to fit your journey. A clear heart and a patient soul yields more power than you could ever imagine."

—*Esther T.*

Detachment

Detachment is powerful. You came here in this physical world by yourself and you will leave this dimension by yourself. When we attach ourselves unnecessarily to people, places, or things of this physical world it hinders our spiritual growth. We aren't meant to be materialistic or attached. We were born for spiritual ascension not worldly attachments. Enjoy everything as is and own things but don't let the things own you. Don't become slaves of things or addicted to people. Your purpose is far higher than you can imagine. These worldly relationships and attachments are your partners on your path to enjoy while they are with you and not to crash down if and when their time is up and they exit. You are on a constant journey of spiritual enlightenment and attainment of your dreams and goals. Enjoy the journey and your fellow travelers on this journey, but don't get attached to anything or anyone.

Experiencing emotions without attachment and their power to control you is detachment. Detach yourself from unnecessary emotions, experiences, and people as their choices, action, and behavior reflect their evolvement and journey. Detachment creates your safe circle of protection. It's your peace & power.

"Remember that there is nothing stable in human affairs, therefore avoid undue elation in prosperity or undie depression in adversity."

—Isocrates

Fear of Future

"If you are feeling frightened about what comes next, don't be. Embrace the uncertainty. Allow it to lead you places. Be brave as it challenges you to exercise both your heart and your mind as you create your own path towards happiness; don't waste time with regret. Spin wildly into your next action. Enjoy the present, each moment, as it comes, because you will never get another one quite like this. And if you should ever look up and find yourself lost, simply take a breath and start over, retrace your steps and go back to the purest place in your heart...where your hope lives. You will find your way again."

—Everwood (TV series)

If you are afraid of sickness, focus on perfect health, if you are afraid of death, focus on eternal life, if you are afraid of failure, focus on success, if you are afraid of poverty, focus on abundance. Face your fears and redirect them towards the exact opposite of what you fear. Alter every fearful thought to a positive exact opposite reality of what you fear and give laser focus and attention to the new thought; slowly your fears will start dissolving.

"Do the thing that you are afraid to do and the death of fear is certain."

—Ralph Waldo Emerson

Relationships

In this life, we will entangle ourselves with numerous souls. There are intimate relationship and then there are relations like family & friends. Each relationship has a purpose on our path. Some stay for longer and some leave sooner. Some provide us with unconditional love, strength, anchor, compassion, and protection and some leave us bitter, angry, and in resentment. Each relationship teaches us something. It's for us to analyze, learn, and involve ourselves accordingly. At times we grow out of people who are not growing.

Compassionate detachment is absolutely necessary if we want our own personal healing and raising our frequencies. Attachment to worldly relations mostly leads to pain; detachment keeps us balanced and strong. We need to focus on ourselves as complete individuals strong enough to take care of ourselves. Worldly relationships are there to enjoy and experience but not to get attached. When we begin to see ourselves as worthy, loveable, abundant, joyful, balanced beings, we attract accordingly.

We have to analyze constantly whether each of our relationships are based on love or fear. Be strong enough to detach yourself from any relationship that does not serve your highest good or is a hindrance to your purpose and path forward.

"In my experience, I have found that the solutions to all of life's intractable problems are not found through any form of intellect or cleverness. They are solved simply by moving on."

—Carl Jung

Staying involved in toxic relationships will deplete us and keep us from moving forward on our soul's advancement journey. We cannot move ahead positively if we continue to allow toxic people to pull us down into the lower vibrational energies of judgments, negativity, sadness, abuse, confusion, chaos, drama, denial, and limited belief systems. Keeping ourselves strongly anchored on the spiritual path and our purpose in life by choosing not to get caught up in relationships that lower our vibrations is not selfish; it actually serves the entire universe.

Choose to live from the pure and sacred source within you and become the director of your own life. Do not allow other people's opinions, criticism, beliefs, actions, reactions, judgments, jealousies & negativities to deter you from living your own authentic divinely aligned purpose and life. Release the people, places, experiences, and events that do not enhance your being, lower your vibrations, or drag you to negativity. Refuse their presence and release any attachment. Your path will be lighter and sacred in positive vibrations.

In personal relationships sometimes one soul elevates to the assigned purpose and raises vibrations accordingly whereas the other soul is still entangled in the lower vibrational aura and refuses to improve or elevate to a better vibrational state. These souls will no longer be a vibrational match and will continue the resistance; hence there will be no harmony amongst them. Usually this is the moment to understand that the particular soul's role in your path is complete and it is time to let go and move forward without them. Give them a chance and guidance to improve and by all means stay in those relationships, if they don't hinder your elevation and you can detach easily. And if they have already left your life, it's a blessing in disguise as they can't go where you are headed.

"Don't worry about the people God removed from your life. He heard conversations you didn't, He saw things you couldn't and He made moves that you wouldn't."

—Anonymous

At the same time when we are on the path of enlightenment and improving ourselves, we feel the souls around us all seem different. We may start judging them too. This is the moment to understand that in this quantum universe anything is possible. All souls are living according to their enlightenment and evolvement. We have no right to judge. We need to let them be. No one is right or wrong. They are at a different level than we are. Higher or lower it doesn't matter. As long as their presence is not toxic to our life, we need to let them be without any judgment. And if their presence is toxic to us then we need to distance ourselves in order to protect our sanity and progression. We have the right to choose who to let in our sacred circle of love and who to distance ourselves from. Everyone brings positive or negative energy. We can feel that and we need to allow accordingly.

Heal your soul by releasing everything that no longer serves purpose in your life and to your highest good and divine energy path. These things include any low vibrational thoughts and beliefs, negativity, pain, toxic relationships, toxic souls, judgments, hurt, or fear. Bless them for their presence, experience, and lesson in your life and set your intentions for new, positive, high vibrational experiences. Release them with love knowing that they have served their purpose and now it's time to move on to a higher vibration; the next level.

Resilience

Resilience is our ability to deal with stress, to respond instead of reacting. There is a deep difference. When you are mentally strong, the stress doesn't change but your ability to deal with it improves. You start responding to things rather than reacting to them. Your flexibility becomes your strength, you learn how to accept and adapt to change. Change is the only constant in life.

"God, give us grace to accept with serenity the things that cannot be changed, Courage to change the things which should be changed and the wisdom to distinguish the one from the other."

—Reinhold Niebuhr

'Wabi-Sabi' is a Japanese concept that explains the beauty of imperfection in this world and the acceptance of change. The resilient soul resists shocks, stress, and negative events and responds to them in peace.

Self-Discipline

Self-discipline is the art of control and direction from temptation to will-power. It is the art of overcoming any weakness and pursuing only that which is of utmost benefit to your mind, body & soul. It is the ability to resist short term temptations for long term beneficial interest. Once you master the art of self-discipline you have the magic key of your personal success in your own hands.

To attain mastery of your life, self-discipline will be the most powerful tool that you can grasp and focus on. It directs your life to always select the best interest for yourself and to achieve balance in every aspect of your being. It gives you strength beyond words when you master this art and apply it to every course of your life. It is the root and foundation of a successful, happy, balanced, and fulfilled life. It takes away the feeling of dependency, addiction, compulsive behavior & temptation.

Take an analysis of your life and write down the areas that you need to work on. Some examples could be procrastination, anger, over-eating, exercise, shopping, gossip, excessive social media browsing, smoking, drinking, over-working, etc. Try and identify the emotions you are trying to fulfill by not having discipline in these areas of your life. The emotions that you are trying to cover up could be anger, fear, unhappiness, resentment, sadness, lack of love, etc. Now take a deep breath and analyze yourself. Isn't this a vicious cycle? No matter how much you shop, or smoke or eat, you end up getting a very short-term high resulting in a severe low, taking you to a lower state than before. This will remain a vicious cycle unless you step up and put an end to this. Take charge! Discipline yourself. I know it's easier said than done. I know this feeling because I have been there for many years of my life. Use this affirmation anytime you are feeling the need to enter your viscous cycle of emotions again

"I am precious and loved. Life is beautiful and the Universe loves me. I am in complete control of myself and my emotions. I have the power to choose my decisions right now. I have the power to direct my emotions in positive alignment. Self-discipline & rituals that I have added in my life bring me power and unlimited strength, directing my course to abundance, prosperity, happiness & success. I am in charge of my life, my thoughts, my emotions, and my actions. I know better now and I will not treat my mind, body, and soul with low vibrational activities. I am the master and I honor myself. I am very precious and I am loved."

Mistakes, Sins & Guilt

We are humans and we all have made mistakes, committed sins, and have deep guilt inside of us which makes some of us to not enjoy life and its beautiful moments. Remember the universe; your sacred source forgives you if you truly, humbly and deeply repent and ask for forgiveness. Learn from your mistakes and make a deep promise to your own soul to never repeat them ever in your life. Release the guilt and ask to be healed and you shall be healed. You don't have to carry the burden, guilt, and weight of your mistakes with you all your life. If you are sacredly aware that it was a mistake and you have truly repented within your soul and learnt the lesson from it to never repeat and hurt anyone again then release this guilt to the universe and ask to be embraced lovingly. Imagine a white light surrounding you and caressing you lovingly. You are safe and loved and your soul is filled with light.

Let go of anything that prevents you to grow mentally physically and emotionally.

Appreciation

Start intentionally appreciating everything that's good around you. Make an effort to thank the universe for things as little as a breeze you feel on your face or the rays of sunshine saturating your face lovingly or a beautiful flower that you see. Appreciate your health, your eyes, and your feet that you walk all day with. When you see your children smile, appreciate their presence, and this gift from the universe. Appreciate your parent's love and presence. Appreciate your partner's love. Appreciate the food that you just ate and the home that you are in.

When you start appreciating you start raising your vibrations and attracting more of what you are appreciating. Your gratitude meditation in the 'SOUL Zone' will help you form this habit. It's a very powerful mantra to activate your manifestation vibration as the universe loves your gratitude state; giving you more and better every time you appreciate. Every moment that you are in gratitude of something, it's a signal to the universe energy to give you more and better.

Healing occurs at the soul level. Your body is just a tool to express the pain. Pain is experienced at the soul state, deeply embedded and your body's condition is just a reaction of that pain. When our heart aches out of hurt or pain it's a signal from your soul to initiate the healing process immediately. Heal at the soul level and your body's condition will automatically improve. Traditional medicines heal or cover the body's condition, Psychotherapy heals the mental mess but you need to go above & beyond by healing your soul. When you heal at the soul level, everything aligns & falls into its perfect place.

Pain from an external worldly source is all part of your karmic lessons & evolvement. Intensely painful experiences like loss of a loved one, tragic incident, destruction, failure of a business or relationship, financial hardship, crisis are all orchestrated events for your life experiences. We have a sacred choice to accept these incidences, feel the emotions & choose to rise above their pain to continue our worldly journey or we can stay in their pain and stagnate our journey taking ourselves to lower vibrations every day. When we choose the latter, we start attracting all experiences and people resonating with lower frequency. You can't control the external worldly circumstances & events but you can control how you respond to them. Rise above their frequency & conquer their negativity with strength, courage & optimism.

Healing Ritual

"My body, mind & soul are created by the Universal Intelligence, the Omnipotent Almighty Power with love. My Source is all wisdom and it knows how to heal me inside out. My Infinite Source has a powerful healing presence within every cell of my body and has initiated the magical process of healing within itself. My body, mind & soul is transforming into a healed, healthy, vivacious, happy, positive state releasing everything that doesn't serve my present and my future. My all-powerful source energy is extracting my fears, my pain, and all my stagnant negative energy and releasing it from my mind, body & soul. It is now saturating every cell of my body with healing light (Nur), love and positivity, raising my vibration to attract, align & Sync with the magnificent universal energy flow. I place deep gratitude in my heart for my 'Source Energy as it heals me and transforms me into a healed light being. I am perfect, I am whole, I am healed, I am loved;

I am an extension of my Source Energy."

Part 3
The 7 Zones

Rituals to transform your mind, body & soul; for a High Vibrational Lifestyle

This is the essence of my last two decades of reading, research, and experiences. I have gone through many rituals to heal myself and rise from the downward spiral I was in and I succeeded eventually. This program is the synopsis of everything that worked for me in healing myself, rising from the downward spiral, and eventually aligning myself to my source energy & achieving my dreams in life. Now I am living the life that syncs with my purpose and it is thanks to all the things that worked for me through trial & error. Now I present you the extract of all the hard work in hope that it will transform your life and help you become the best version of yourself; assisting you to attaining your ultimate destiny.

I always thought that happy, healthy, successful people had something that the ordinary people did not have. In fact my years of research proved me wrong. The extraordinary souls had nothing special and different than the ordinary. They just 'CHOSE' to live their life differently following certain rituals, making certain lifestyle choices that eventually ended them up with success, health, vitality, and ultimately their dream life.

The steps that help you achieve your optimum life are very simple. Nothing too hard to follow but they require commitment and consistency. I promise you with experience that if you commit to achieving your high vibrational lifestyle you will be rewarded with happiness, health, vitality, abundance, and financial freedom. If you incorporate these 7 zones in your day, you will heal yourself and achieve everything that you ever dreamt of in your life. If you plan your day making sure these 7 zones are taken care of in your daily life then nothing can stop you from achieving your optimum life.

I can say with utmost confidence that this 'ZONE plan' is the best synopsis that I can present to you. It is the essence of my entire life efforts to find the practical and doable methodologies that work. Over the years of accumulating information and testing various things to achieve optimum results for the high vibrational lifestyle, the 'ZONE plan' is the extract of everything that has worked for me, presented in a concise and planned manner so it's simple to follow. I have taken the guesswork out of living your optimum life and devised a plan that is simple, transparent & result-based.

The benefits of following this plan would yield in:

- Raising your vibration
- Success in personal & financial life
- Healing of your mind, body & soul
- Increased energy and mental clarity
- Happiness & the drive to live life to the fullest
- Achieving your perfect health & weight
- Attainment of your optimum mind state
- Aid in fighting disease in your body
- Anti-aging and optimum skin health
- Longevity boosting
- Rejuvenating your entire system to optimum level
- Positive thought process

"Successful people are simply those with successful habits."

—Brian Tracy

It's the formula that millions of people already follow in one aspect or the other and the ones who follow these things daily in their lives have proven to succeed without limits. You can be that person if you commit to yourself today. The moment is now. Commit to healing yourself and taking yourself to the optimum level that you can achieve by following these steps and living life to the fullest.

"You will never change your life until you change something you do daily. The secret of your success is found in your daily routine."

—Annie Dillard

This is your life and the fact that you have this book in your hands is an affirmation that the universe is on your side helping you to get up, raise yourself from this dark place and achieve the best; prioritize yourself. If you are suffering from:

- Low energy
- Negativity
- Sadness
- Anxiety
- Depression
- Overthinking
- Procrastination
- Pressure
- Self-criticism
- Fear
- Feeling of helplessness
- Stagnant state of life
- Emotional outbreak
- Weight issues
- Stress
- Feeling of being lost
- Financial instability
- Tiredness
- Skin health issues
- Relationship issues

- Suicidal thoughts
- Low self-esteem

I want you to know that you are not alone. I suffered from almost all these things listed above and I recovered myself. You have hope and you can heal and come back to life. I will help you recover and heal. If I can come out of that dark place and achieve everything I ever wanted, so can you. I'm no different than you. All I did was commit to myself. I was tired of being in the low vibrational state.

"The meaning of life is to find your gift; the purpose of life is to give it away."

—William Shakespeare

Why am I so intensely in the state to help you? Because I have been there and I know how it feels to be in that state. I found my purpose by going through all my trials and here I am giving all my knowledge to you. This is the moment I have been waiting for all my life; to fulfill my purpose; to help and heal you! I promise you that whatever state you are in right now, if you incorporate the following 7 ZONES in your life; you will achieve anything you want.

You may be in a very low state in life as of right now wanting to heal, recover and rise or you may be in a good state wanting to rise from wherever you are to your optimum. Whichever the case, aligning your life from here onwards to the following zones will change your life. Let's take this moment to analyze where you are in life. Your choices, your decisions, your daily schedule, your words, your thoughts, your actions, your reactions, your finances, your relationships, your mental state, your physical being, your hearts wavelength and take this moment to tell yourself that from this day onwards you will stop perishing and start growing & living.

"What greater wealth is there than to own your life and to spend it on growing? Every living thing must grow. It can't stand still. It must grow or perish."

—Ayan Rand (Atlas Shrugged)

What will you choose?

Let's stop perishing and let's start growing every single moment of our upcoming days, months, and years; till our last breath on this earth. When you wake up every morning you have a choice to grow or perish. What you chose to do that particular day defines if you grew or perished that particular day. Chose to grow; chose to live!

"In order to become the 1%, you must do what the other 99% won't!"

—Anonymous

Have you ever seen a happy, healthy, successful individual making these choices?

- Eating fast-food daily & eating to feed emotions
- Sleeping very late and waking up miserable
- Not working out and living a very sedentary lifestyle
- Always running to get things done in a mechanical vicious circle
- Financially unstable never being able to make ends meet
- Shopping excessively to fill the void
- Thinking negative things all day and repeating sad moments in mind
- Picking low vibration foods at the grocery store
- Talking negatively about people
- Not reading

"The secret of change is to focus all of your energy, not on fighting the old, but on building the new."

—Socrates

Where you are right now is a result of who you were, your habits, your choices, your decisions, and your actions. Where you will be a few years from now will be a result entirely on who you choose to be from this moment onwards. Decide if you want to be at this state or better and take a step towards committing your life to reach your optimum self hence your highest vibration;

resulting in the most healthy, happy, and successful life for yourself. Your daily habits determine the success of your dreams. What you do daily becomes your life. The habits and your daily routine are the secret to your success and destiny. It is as simple as that; if you desire an extraordinary life, you must be on the path of becoming an extraordinary person so you can attract and create your life and be a magnet to peace, happiness, abundance & success. Through my intensive research, I have formulated these 7 Zones that you should be focusing on every single day in order to be on the path of high vibrational lifestyle and eventually manifesting your dreams.

Progression of the mind, body & soul is an accumulation of improving several aspects of your life; hence the collection of the 7 Zones targeting the 7 key areas of our lives and their vibrational ascension.

"The secret of your future is hidden in your daily routine."

—Mike Murdock

When you start your day, there is no future and there is no past, there is only the present moment, the present day, how you live that day determines how you shape your future. When you intentionally take charge of your habits, your 7 Zones, and your day; your life miraculously falls into place in the most magnificent manner. Every single day is a re-birth, it is your chance to live this day like there is no tomorrow. Begin each day with the most brilliant smile and energy. As soon as you open your eyes, smile, and thank the universe for another day of your life. Start every single day with a smile, a goal, discipline, and powerful positive energy and you will notice that the day responds to you in the same manner. The frequency that you radiate will receive the same reaction from the universe. I'm not saying you will never be faced by problems; they will always be there but your attitude towards them will change. How you approach, handle, and respond to them will change miraculously; hence transforming you into a strong soul.

"We are what we repeatedly do. Excellence, then, is not an act, but a habit."

—Will Durant (The Story of Philosophy)

The goal is to achieve excellence through repetition of the rituals that enhance you inside out and become the tool for your growth. The secret lies in focusing on yourself and incorporating these 7 Zones in your day effortlessly; resulting in your time, energy, and attention being spent towards your growth and ultimately taking you to manifest your dreams into reality. The key is to understanding that it's not the timings as much as the mindset that matters. Your mind-set every single morning and throughout the day will shape your day; and ultimately your life. It is a well-known fact that almost all self-made entrepreneurs and successful individuals have a few key things in their life; discipline, focus & routine. Almost all of them are early-risers and use this fantastic golden hour to interact with the universe and in return achieve everything they have ever wanted. Waking up with a smile and purpose changes everything.

"You will never change your life until you change something you do daily. The secret of your success is found in your daily routine."

—John C. Maxwell

Have you noticed how your average day goes? If you calculate intentionally how much time is wasted on mindless browsing on social media or negative thoughts, you'll be shocked. The 7 Zones is an intentional utilization of your time into aspects that will enhance your growth and improve you every single minute of your day directing you towards your purpose and dreams. We all have the same number of hours in a day to spend, yet some of us waste them ruthlessly. It's not the issue of time, its first of all lack of direction and secondly a decision of priority.

"Lack of direction, not Lack of time, is the problem. We all have twenty-four hours days."

—Zig Ziglar

Commit yourself to incorporating these 7 Zones in your life as these will build a very strong foundation in your life yielding massive results. This will require extraordinary levels of commitment and discipline. If you follow through these 7 zones for the next 7 weeks of your life, you will find yourself transforming into the committed and disciplined individual who will be on the path to extraordinary levels of personal, professional & financial success you have always dreamt of. These zones will elevate you to a level so you can elevate your quality of life and achieve success. This will reprogram your entire system to become the greatest powerhouse to attract only the best and high vibrational energy for prosperity, abundance, success, happiness and peace. These Zones will take you from ordinary to extraordinary.

"People don't decide their future. They decide their habits and their habits decide their future."

—F. M. Alexander

Unwavering faith and extraordinary efforts create miracles. And these zones will direct you towards this. Upgrade your day by following these 7 zones and incorporating these rituals and will upgrade your life miraculously. Where you are now is a result of the habits you chose previously, but where you will be in the next few years depends entirely on your choices and decisions about your day & life from this moment onwards. Few years from now your life will be the direct result of the result of who you've become following these 7 zones.

7 weeks of commitment, focus & alignment can place you 7 years ahead in your life. Commitment, focus & consistency are powerful tools to achieve anything that you desire. Prioritize yourself.

The Soul Zone

We have isolated ourselves completely from the 'Infinite Intelligence', 'God', 'The Universe', and 'The Eternal Almighty'. We are so engrossed in the daily mechanical system of this worldly life that we have unplugged ourselves from the earth, its vibrations, frequency, energy, and it's light. We are surrounded by technology, electronic gadgets, day to day issues, work and life and we are in the vicious never-ending cycle which has turned us into stressed, tired, depressed, sad, and empty souls.

It is time to reconnect to our roots and the vibrations of earth. Syncing back to the universal energy is our only way to achieve calmness, serenity, peace, happiness, and take ourselves out of this mechanical daily routine that we are in. When we make an effort to reconnect with the universe, we will begin to see how our life starts becoming more meaningful as we progress towards high vibrations. When we sync back to our roots, we will see how the entire universe rushes to our assistance and guidance for everything in our life. We will never feel alone and sad, we will have the entire universe working besides us, for us.

We have all come to this sad conclusion that this world around us is a final reality whereas it's the exact opposite. This world is a bridge that we are passing through from one dimension to another. We are in physical form for a very short time frame and our eternal reason of being has nothing to do with our daily mechanical life. We have a much higher purpose that we are completely ignoring hence running our days like sad overworked stressed machines. The real purpose of us is constant connection with our infinite intelligence, the universe, 'God', our subconscious mind, and progression to the higher vibrations through everyday beautiful vital rituals that improve us from inside out and raise our vibrations automatically.

We are part of the earth energy and the universal frequency. When we think of ourselves as a separate entity; our frequency doesn't sync creating all sorts of blockages. Aligning ourselves back to our roots is the key to fulfillment.

When we align to our universal energy our day to day lives become poetic and simple. The whole rush just disappears, calmness overtakes the chaos, and finally, we feel we are home as that's where we actually belong.

This zone is about healing your deep inner self and improving your connection with the universe. This is the most important zone of all as this is the root of alignment. The rituals enhanced in this zone will create a strong foundation in your life-sustaining your strength and improving your inner self to a miraculous degree. When you incorporate the rituals defined in this zone in your daily life you will build a very intense foundation for yourself connected to the universe in the deepest level possible. This will make your daily life a source of joy & tranquility. You will start handling life in the calmest and most beautiful manner. You will have the strength to handle stress and worldly problems. You will be amazed at the kind of person you will transform into. Your soul will be at constant peace-giving you the stability to handle life and directing you to the best pathway for your goals.

Starting each day with moments of calmness, silence and tranquility will reduce your stress levels immediately and assist you in starting your day with a clear mind; helping you to take on everything with focus, clarity, calmness, and peace. Enhancing your 'Soul Zone' is a very strong pathway to raise your vibrations and connect your energy with the ultimate frequency of the earth & ultimately the universe. You can achieve this by incorporating some or all of these rituals below in your daily life. These soul enhancing rituals include:

- Breathing
- Prayer
- Affirmations
- Visualization
- Gratitude
- Meditation

- Sound healing
- Journaling
- Nature
- Protection

If you choose not to change your habits and Lifestyle, you are intentionally selecting your current lifestyle & habits; hence your life will be exactly where you are now in the coming years.

Breathing

When we arrived in this world, the first thing we all did, was take a breath; and the last moment we will have on this earth will be defined by our last breath. Breathing is life; life is breaths. We inhale & exhale every single moment unconsciously. Close your eyes for a few seconds and pay attention to your breathing; inhale & exhale. This is your life in these moments. Now take this moment to feel the vitality of the term 'Breathing'. We inhale and that ritual sends oxygen to every single cell of our body to perform its function. We exhale and release the unwanted energy from our system. We are taking a blessing from the universe with every single breath. What a beautiful gift we receive every moment.

"With every breath, you are adding to your life and with every out-breath you are releasing what is not contributing to your life. Every breath is a re-birth."

—Allan Rufus

How to get into an immediate calm state; your happy zone

Inhale for 3 seconds (from your nose)

Hold for 5 seconds

Exhale for 7 seconds (From your mouth)

Repeat till you smile

Repeat this serene ritual for a few times and notice your body's energy changing. You will feel your body coming alive and your energy will be calmer. When we consciously breathe, we become one with the universe, we bring ourselves to the power of the present moment. We clear our mind from all thoughts and bring that moment from the past or future to the beauty of the present. Breathing deeply and consciously for a few minutes everyday readjusts our system and syncs us back to our natural alignment. These simple rituals aid in raising our vibrations and helps release our body, mind, and soul from negativity. Fill your body with deep breaths and it will fill you with peace. Mornings and evening, take a few moments to consciously breathe and start seeing the transformation of your soul zone.

"Breath is the bridge which connects life to consciousness, which unites your body to your thoughts. Whenever your mind becomes scattered, use your breath as the means to take hold of your mind again."

—Thich Nhat Hanh

Prayer

Praying is the most beautiful form of communication with the universe. It may have a religious connotation to some but realistically it's just a precious moment between you and the ultimate entity. A moment of surrender, peace & belonging. A tranquil ritual where you close your eyes and speak softly to the universe. Every morning I start my day with a moment of prayer. I close my eyes and take this enchanted ritual as my quality time with my 'Creator'. I speak about love, peace, serenity, and dreams. I ask about guidance & strength. I thank you for all the miracles in my life and ask for more. It's an absolutely miraculous few minutes of my morning where I have a one on one moment with the ultimate frequency. This blesses my day in the most magnificent manner.

"Knock, And He'll open the door. Vanish, And He'll make you shine like the sun. Fall, And He'll raise you to the heavens. Become nothing, And He'll turn you into everything."

—Rumi

Praying is a magnificent medium that fills our soul with the divine love from our 'Creator', our divine omnipotent source. When we pray we fill our spirit with loving light and this light loves, and protects us beyond measure. We elevate our soul to a beautiful divine aura when we pray. Praying calms our soul and nourishes it intensely with sacred light. Praying lights up our entire being. Prayer is a sacred ritual that aligns us directly with our source energy. Create a special area for this ritual. I have a beautiful small rug, a cushion, candles, and my mala beads in a serene corner in my room. I call it my blessed corner. Always remember that your thoughts are your silent prayers. Be extremely guarded with your thoughts as silent prayers are answered regardless; as they are prayers after all.

"And though thy knees were never bent,

To heaven thy hourly prayers are sent,

And Whether formed for good or ill

Are registered and answered still."

—Ralph Waldo Emerson (Prayer)

Pray for others

Imagine a white light radiating from you towards the entire humanity and the universe. Pray that you are a source of love, inspiration, blessings, and service to others. Pray that everyone around you is radiating with love, healing, prosperity, and abundance. When you pray for others, the blessings are reflected back in your life in abundance.

"I find it really beautiful when someone prays for you without you knowing. I don't think there is any form of deeper, purer love."

—Anonymous

Affirmations

Your thoughts and words play such a vital role in your life. What you say to yourself becomes your reality. If you want to improve your life and your mind-set, you must affirm positivity daily. When you repeat the positive words to yourself every day, your subconscious mind starts to accept them and your life starts changing. Affirmations help to upgrade your thoughts, your mind, and your life. The right way to introduce affirmations in your daily life is vital. The right affirmations boost your life in a miraculous way. When they are done the right way and daily as a meaningful ritual in your life, they connect to your subconscious at a very deep level enhancing and improving your mindset resulting in your conscious mind to elevate your vibrations.

It's a chain reaction that starts with positivity of words and ends in positivity of life events.

Daily Affirmations help with your commitment to action. Discipline, focus, and commitment are the keys to success with all the rituals explained in this book. You can't get something just by wanting it but you can get that thing by your desire, focus, rituals, and commitment. Write your affirmations down and closely study them, then next to each affirmation write down the necessary actions you will take to reach your goals. This will give you clarity and provide pathway to your dreams. Your affirmations should be specific and result oriented. Affirmations can be about all areas of your life that you would like to change or improve, health, personal, financial, parenting, relationships, etc. As you grow in life the specific areas that you need to improve and work on will change accordingly.

Affirmation Examples

Example 1: *I am going to nourish my body the right way so I can heal and achieve my body's optimum state providing the right quality nutrients to my body.*

Plan of Action: I am devoting myself to lead a healthy holistic lifestyle and improve my eating habits. I am dedicated to incorporating superfoods in my life and avoid fast foods. I will commit myself to cook at home at least three days a week and prepare my lunches so I can avoid fast foods and binge eating. I will go for a walk daily for 20 min in the morning to jump-start my day with physical exercise. I am giving myself 90 days for this goal and I will achieve it as this will ensure my direction towards my goals and will raise my vibration.

Example 2: *I am going to increase my income three times so I can be on the path to financial freedom and increase the quality of my lifestyle; living financially stress-free days.*

Plan of Action: I am devoting myself to additional certifications to enhance my skills. I am dedicated to initiating my online business that I have been planning. I will commit myself to one hour every day for certifications and one hour for setting up my online business. I will stop procrastinating and invest this time for my financial security, committing myself to two hours a day for my income enhancement. I am giving myself 120 days for this goal and I will achieve it as this will ensure my direction towards my goals and will raise my vibration.

Example 3: *I am going to start writing the book that I have been thinking about so I can feel the accomplishment that I desire intensely. It's been a lifelong dream and this is the right time to start working on it.*

Plan of Action: I am devoting myself to waking up a bit earlier than usual and spending one hour of my morning on this dream. I am dedicated to writing 350 words every day. I will commit myself to spend this time 5 days a week as it will turn into my book within 6 months of this dedication. 350 words x 5 days is 1750 words a week and 1750 words x 26 weeks is 45500 words, hence an entire book completed within 6 months of dedication. I will stop procrastinating and start investing this time for my lifelong dream, committing myself to one hour a day, five days a week for my goal. I am giving myself 26 weeks for this goal and I will achieve it as this will ensure my direction towards my success and will raise my vibration.

Example 4: *I am going to be a source of love and healing to make a difference in this world and leave every person that I meet better than I found them.*

Plan of Action: I am devoting myself to radiating love and compassion from my being. I am dedicated to sincerely making a difference in every soul that I encounter in my day. I will look at every person with extreme kindness and compassion, without judgment. I will commit myself to honor the person's soul and use my words to enhance their lives. I am giving myself 30 days for this goal and I will achieve it as this will ensure my direction towards my goals and will raise my vibration.

Synopsis

These are a few examples of the right way to invest in 'Affirmations'. There is a strategy behind these written statements with a pattern of goals and steps for achievement. They reprogram your subconscious mind to focus its attention towards your goals and direct your mind towards everything that will help you to achieve them. Always say things in a positive connotation; Instead of "I don't want to be financially unstable "; say "I want to be financially stable". Use positive words; as this will result in your conscious mind keeping you focused towards your priorities directing you towards taking the actions necessary to accomplish your goals. You write your goals and you write the steps that you will take to be in the right direction to reach your goals. This will give you clarity, focus, routine, and direction. The more specific and detail-oriented your affirmations are, the clearer your subconscious mind will absorb it and start working on it.

When you read your affirmations daily, in a positive state feeling as if they have already happened, your life will take a positive turn towards your purpose and dreams. Read every single affirmation with strong feelings of determination, positivity, and excitement. Every ritual will lead you towards finding your purpose and achieving your ultimate destiny. Review your goals and affirmations every few months to make sure of their validity in your life. You may check off some goals with your dedication, you may add affirmations every once in a while. This is an ongoing ritual in your life which will be added and improved periodically as your life changes and your vibrations rise.

Visualization

Visualization is a very powerful technique by which you use your imagination to create an actual image in your mind of exactly how you want a particular event, person, or thing to be in your future. It is an extremely mystical, spiritual and miraculous ritual that is proven to give results if you perform it the right way. It has long been a practice used by people to enhance their performance and achieve results. It trains your mind to take your thoughts and convert them into words, pictures, experiences, and emotions. It provides you with the feeling of experiencing exactly how you want your future to be, hence making your dreams turn into a reality.

"Having seen and felt the end, you have willed the means to the realization of the end."

—Thomas Troward

Visualization works in an enchanting manner. Your intentional thoughts turn into an image with feelings and this in turn becomes your reality. Our mind cannot tell the difference between an actual experience and a vivid visualization. Hence our continuous act of visualization with emotions embeds in our subconscious mind as an actual experience, attracting to us all experiences, people, and things accordingly. For pure and powerful visualization, we have to let go of certain emotions like guilt, fear, the thought that we are not worth it, not adequate enough, not capable enough, and not lucky enough.

The best time for visualization is after your affirmations, as this is the moment of clarity and calmness. You are already in alignment with source after your meditation and affirmations, your visualization ritual will be extremely powerful at this time. For this ritual start with a feeling of calmness and let all feelings of doubt, fear, limitations, negativity or sadness leave your aura. Initiate this ritual with extreme positivity, faith, strength, and peace. Take yourself in a state of magic and enchantment where logic and limits do not exist as this is the actual source aura. Now start visualizing exactly what you want and how you want it. Feel your visualization as it's happening 'NOW'. Involve all your senses; see, smell, feel, touch, and taste every single detail of your current visualized state. The more real and vivid your visualization will be; the more strongly it will embed in your subconscious mind as reality. This enhances your guidance towards achieving your goals.

To experience the highest intensity results of successful visualization is to imagine yourself in real and flawless execution of your goals in your visualization. This is an extremely powerful ritual in overcoming any limitations you have in your mind.

When you combine meditation with gratitude, affirmations, and visualization, you activate a powerful state of your mind, body, and soul, turbo-charging your subconscious mind to guide your conscious mind for high-intensity performance; resulting in achievement and success.

Imagine as if your goals have been achieved and now visualize your life. Create experiences in your mind with the strong belief that your dreams have already manifested. Imagine yourself living in your dream home, visualize yourself in your new bedroom overlooking the sea, watching the sunset, and savor every moment as it's already happening. Imagine signing your book in your favorite book store, cherishing the feeling of accomplishment on the publishing of your dream book. Imagine driving inside your favorite car taking turns and reminiscing the gorgeous landscape around, the cool breeze caressing your face. Imagine yourself in your favorite country walking around savoring the architecture and people around you. Visualize your dreams as they have already manifested. Visualize with emotions, faith, and belief, then watch them manifesting in reality right in front of your eyes.

Gratitude

Gratitude is a miracle mantra that attracts unlimited positivity. When you radiate the frequency of gratitude, the universe gives you ten folds of the same in return. It's a simple yet strong phenomenon of attracting abundance, happiness, serenity, and peace. When you are thankful you are in a state of bliss and tranquility; this gives the universe a signal to give you more of what you are thankful for, to give you more of what you want to keep you in that state. When you give something to someone and they are extremely thankful to you, you immediately go in the state of happiness. The same formula occurs with the universe. When the universe gets into the "Givers" state and is appreciated, it wants to give more; it's a natural phenomenon and law of universe.

Whatever you have, be grateful for it. Being grateful allows you to raise your vibration and attract even better things into your life. Negative events in your life can help you awaken and become a better person. Be grateful for everything that has happened in your life, because everything happens for a reason. Whether it is a lesson or a blessing, it brought something into your life and ultimately changed you for the better. Open your receiving channel. We have been programmed and trained to give and not receive. We have been instilled with the perception that receiving is somehow selfish. That's not true; when you express gratitude and open your receiving channels you attract everything that's meant for you.

This is the most beautiful 'Gratitude Ritual' that I learnt from Abraham-Hicks Teachings and it's an honor to share it. Look towards the sky outside and take this moment to acknowledge and thank you're the universe for everything.

"I acknowledge and accept the existence of your love and that I am the focus of your worthy, beneficial, and positive awareness. I appreciate and love your constant focus, attention, and love for my wellbeing and dreams. I take this moment of my present and thank that you are with me,

- *Protecting me*
- *Appreciating me*
- *Loving me*
- *Healing me*
- *Uplifting me*
- *Guiding me*
- *Granting me*
- *Assisting me*
- *Acknowledging me*
- *Supporting me*
- *Helping me*
- *Showing me*
- *Easing me*
- *Leading me*
- *Taking me towards my dreams*

I thank you for your unconditional positive love, guidance, and grants, for all you are and all you do. I am blessed, I am worthy, I am ready, I allow myself to receive, and I am ready to receive more and more from you with love and happiness." (inspired from Abraham-Hicks Teachings)

Meditation

Meditation is the fastest and purest way to raise your vibrations as the real you is not the physical being that you think you are; it is the energy, the spirit, and the soul. Prayer and meditation both are beautiful forms of raising your aura and connecting to your sacred source energy. Prayer combined with meditation and gratitude is a powerful healing combination that takes your energy to an extremely divine state.

Meditating daily is a powerful ritual. It literally draws your sacred source energy towards you as you silence your mind to focus on your source. Just a few minutes a day can initiate tremendous results. It realigns your energy within your body strengthening your connection with your source. It quiets your mind and stills your thought process hence giving you the ability to listen to your scared self; your source energy. It allows your soul to connect to your higher self and receive the goldmine of information being released for you constantly in order to reach your destiny. You need this moment of stillness and silence to be able to receive the divine information that is being released to your benefit.

Meditation calms your nerves and gives you clarity. Your thoughts entangle your mind 24/7 consciously and sub-consciously. Silencing your mind enables you to open your heart and detect the valuable messages being sent to you by your source. It helps you in programming your subconscious mind to guide you better to reach your destiny.

"There is a force within which gives you life, seek that!

In your heart lies a priceless gem; seek that.

O wandering soul, if you want to

find the greatest treasure, don't look outside,

look inside and seek that."

—Rumi

Meditation is a gift that will reprogram your subconscious mind and will connect you with yourself and the universe. It is an extremely powerful ritual for transformation. There are many ways to meditate and many different kinds of meditations. You can look for guided meditations online and follow them if you have never tried meditation before. Initially, it may not be easy to meditate but slowly you will get used to this beautiful ritual as it takes you to a serene state. You can meditate about your success and dreams, your perfect health and wellbeing, the love of your life, or more. Always look at yourself lovingly when you are meditating. Self-love is extremely vital to heal yourself. Meditation can be anywhere from 5 minutes to an hour depending on the time you have and the rituals intensity.

Meditation Ritual

Find a quiet comfortable place, outside or inside. Sit comfortably or lay down, begin by focusing on your breath. Inhale and exhale deeply, focus on being in the now.

Try and slowly bring your thought to a halt, there is no past or future, just this moment.

Continue following your breath inhaling positivity and exhaling all negativity.

Close your eyes and imagine yourself in a serene place, feel peaceful and now start imagining how you would like your life ideally to be, your dreams, your passion, your goals and your happiness.

Now feel and imagine that you are already living that life. Continue breathing in and out. Feel the wind, savor the beautiful surroundings.

Feel and connect to this moment and enjoy living your dream. Spend a few minutes here cherishing and living every moment how you want it.

Once you are fully immersed, enjoy the serenity and intensity of this new reality that you are consciously co-creating with your subconscious mind.

Now slowly bring yourself back to the room that you are in.

Keep breathing in and out.

Repeat every day to align yourself to the universe

Two Powerful Meditations

Evening Meditation

- Another beautiful day has come to an end and the moments of rejuvenation, relaxation, tranquility, peace, calmness, serenity and rest surrounds me now.
- I thank the 'Almighty', 'The Eternal source' for this successful day. I did everything to the best of my ability and will attract the best results.
- I surrender and release ego, control, and fear; asking my source to merge with me for my highest good.
- I release all stress and negative emotions that may have surrounded me and I end my day with love and serenity.
- My utmost faith is in the 'Divine power' that is the creator of all things and this faith that I have is my sacred treasure and fortune.
- I lived this day with happiness and positive expectations and only positivity comes towards me.
- All my thoughts are the epitome of optimism, abundance, goodness, happiness, peace, tranquility, and prosperity.
- *I take this moment of quietness and relaxation to place sacred seeds of positive*

thoughts in my subconscious mind. Thoughts of pure love, prosperity, calmness, abundance, wealth, spiritual growth, success, happiness, security, freedom, and tranquility are entering my sacred subconscious mind and embedding themselves in every cell of my body. I am a part of the universe's eternal love and light so all my thoughts are reaching my eternal source for them to become my reality. I am syncing back to where I belong and I am blessed.

- The glory, magnificence, and supremacy of universe's love will be expressed through me, blessing me now, always and forever.

- I affirm and acknowledge with love that there is an unlimited source and it's the principle of life. Every single thing in this universe is created by the 'Omnipotent' and flows through it. I am blessed to be the loving focus of the 'Supreme Magnificence' with abundance in every way flowing towards me.

- I allow myself to receive all this abundance now and forever. I have become a channel of abundance, prosperity, happiness, beauty, healing, and peace and this flows through me for humanity to be blessed; through my choices and creative avenues.

- I am ready to receive and give. I am ready to be the recipient and the giver to be part of the endless flow of this universe.

- I am in harmony with the flow of this universe and its infinite eternal abundance.
- All these thoughts are embedding in my subconscious mind, syncing into my being and will be reflected in my life from this moment onwards.
- The 'Sacred Nur' (Gods Light) is surrounding my aura protecting me. The same light is surrounding my home and my loved ones protecting and shielding them, radiating with love.
- Infinite Intelligence is guiding me and directing my life to the best.
- I defy all evil and negativity and refuse to accept their presence around me as I acknowledge that they are illusions. I don't deny their presence; I just don't want their presence around my aura.
- I have complete faith that every circumstance, event, or person coming my way is aligned with my purpose.
- I know that my sole purpose in this life is to align myself with the infinite intelligence and move upward and outward expanding my being to sync with the universe's magical frequency.
- The 'Infinite Intelligence', my subconscious mind, 'The Almighty' is all 'ONE' and independent of space and time. It can leave my body, travel to any place at any time and any dimension to bring me

exactly the event and circumstance beneficial to my desire and dreams.

- I release the limitations, lack, and inhibitions of my past. It's my sacred genesis now and every day of my life from this moment onwards is advancement towards my source. I am guided, loved, healed, and blessed.

- When I call upon my source, I become 'ONE' with its powers and align with all its wisdom and intelligence guiding and directing my day and my life till my last breath.

- Every desire, dream, and goal that I have is guided and answered from this perfect infinite limitless, inexhaustible source of wisdom, power, and abundance.

Morning Meditation

- I wake up to this beautiful day and the following years of my life with a radiant smile, gratitude, happiness, peace, serenity, and abundance.

- I'm radiating Nur (God's Light) through me. I am healthy, happy, joyous, and beaming with the glory of the Infinite love. The 'Universe', 'God', 'Infinite Intelligence' is all-powerful and the source of all amenities in my life.

- I ask and intend to connect with my sacred loving source and I allow myself to receive the loving and healing light continuously and effortlessly reaching every cell in my body empowering it and alleviating it to the highest scared vibrations.

- I'm saying these words to engrave these thoughts in my infinitely intelligent subconscious mind which is the epitome of abundance and is the source of everything.

- I detach myself from all negative thoughts, experiences, people, events, or vibrations. I know that they are just illusions and I don't accept their presence around me. I surround myself with sacred, positive, happy, peaceful, prosperous vibrations, light, and energy.

- I accept all divine abundance, wealth, happiness, peace, and health to flow to me with the pure divine love and blessings. Abundance flows effortlessly, ceaselessly, and joyously in my experience.

- Eternal sacred glorious omnipotent love, natural spiritual law and supreme order governs my life through the eternal sacred divine love.

- I surround myself with Nur (Gods Light) and let it enter my being reaching every cell in my body radiating sacred presence and love through me.

- I can flow into my experience whatever I desire, want, or need.
- *I see myself surrounded by all who are in the same vibration as I am with only positive thoughts and growth mindset; with pure intentions and sacred aura. With unlimited abundance and prosperity, with happiness, clarity, calmness, and peace, appreciating each other's success and desires; praying for each other.*
- I am in perfect health in this physical life experience. Every cell in my body is alive and healthy radiating love and happiness.
- I am accessing power of the unlimited universe through the power of allowing and power of attraction.
- The sacred eternal source is available to me through the 'Law of Attraction', 'Law of Allowing', 'Law of Receiving', 'Law of Abundance', and the 'Law of Opulence'. I allow all these laws to work for me and flow through me effortlessly.
- I am birthed in this physical dimension to be a source of help to humanity, to succeed, to experience the 'Infinite Intelligence' work with me and through me for my highest good and with pure intentions.

- Supreme security and protection surround me with a glorious white light. I am loved, nurtured, protected, and shielded.
- Sacred peace fills my soul, eternal love encompasses my heart and mind.' Infinite Supreme Omnipotent Intelligence' guides me every day of my life. All glorious riches and abundance of this 'Supreme Almighty's' power and wealth flows to me effortlessly and endlessly.
- I am advancing forward every single day expanding my horizons physically, emotionally, mentally, spiritually, and financially. From this moment onwards every second of my life will be towards growth, abundance, flow of love, and infinite advancement.
- I acknowledge the 'Almighty', 'Universe', and 'Eternal Supreme' and I acknowledge that it is my eternal source of everything that I want, need, or desire.
- I acknowledge that I am the focal point and the love of this source and it is constantly beaming and radiating towards me fulfilling every desire I have in this moment, space, and time.
- I am aligned perfectly with my source now to allow and receive everything in abundance, prosperity, love, health, peace, tranquility, wealth, spirituality, and luck. It is flowing to me in eternal abundance.

- My 'Supreme Scared Source' will multiply all that is coming my way and all that I have in million folds according to the infinite sources.
- My eternal sacred source constantly guides me for the best and reveals to me my purpose so I can be a source of blessing to humanity.
- I trust the wisdom and intelligence of the 'Almighty' and the 'Source' within and allow it to guide me forever for the best of my interest.

Healing & Raising Your Vibrations with Sounds

'Sound Healing' is an ancient ritual, which dates back to ancient Greece, when music was used to heal different ailments. Healing with sounds has numerous health benefits, including immune system improvement, lowered stress levels, decreasing anxiety, lowering blood pressure, pain reduction, promoting relaxation, enhancing focus, improving sleep quality, and raising your vibrational frequency. This is an ancient ritual which is still used in modern era for healing & relaxation. Sound is vibrations measured by their frequency. Frequency is the number of vibrations or sound waves per second and is measured in Hz (Hertz). Every sound around us is energy & vibrations. The words we speak are also sound and its energy.

Sound Healing from Earthly Solfeggio Frequencies

Grounding & Centering – 174 Hz

Creation & Creativity – 258 Hz

Freedom & Liberation – 396 Hz

Soul Transformation – 417 Hz

Love & Passion – 528 Hz

Spiritual Empowerment – 639 Hz

Creating Sacred Space – 741 Hz

Intuitive Awareness – 852 Hz

An example is the 528 Hz frequency. It is the most significant of the ancient Solfeggio Frequencies. It's known as the 'Miracle' frequency or the 'Love' frequency. It is strongly rooted with nature found in human DNA and Chlorophyll. It is identified as the mathematical matrix of the universe and has proven healing potential. This frequency has a spiritual & earthly connection in the Solfeggio Scale.

Everything around us is energy, frequency, vibration & waves. Sound healing uses the exact methodology to induce relaxation by syncing our frequency to the particular healing sound frequency. When sound waves reach our ears, they are received by our nerves in the part of the brain that processes sound. Once they reach our brain, they trigger the specific level of frequency to sync. This process also alters our emotional state accordingly, releasing particular hormones & triggering emotions as per the desired frequency.

Listening to sounds fills our brain with dopamine & releases oxytocin, which is a natural painkiller. There are different types of sound healings and you can choose what syncs best with you. There is 'Binaural Sounds', 'Multidimensional music', 'Psych geometric music', 'Tibetan Singing Bowls', 'Sonic

Acupuncture', 'Shamanism, Healing' with voice & the 'Taoist Technique' amongst a few. Personally, 'The Binaural Beats' is what works for me. They synchronize the brain giving clarity, concentration & alertness. There are different frequency levels for different purposes, such as 'Beta', 'Alpha', 'Theta', and 'Delta'. Include the sounds in your daily meditation, your walks, creative zones & evening rituals and they will activate healing & raise your frequency.

Journaling

Writing what you want or feel gives you enormous clarity & programs your subconscious mind towards a certain unified clear goal. Journaling is a very common habit amongst many successful individuals. A consistent habit of writing your feelings, your aspirations, your goals & dreams is a crucial part of conveying the message to your subconscious self as to exactly what you would like to achieve. Once your subconscious starts getting the clear messages it directs you towards the exact ways & means required for you to fulfill your destiny. Your soul zone is the perfect time to incorporate 10-15 minutes of journaling every day.

Write about your dreams & exactly how you would like your life to be. Write about your goals and everything you have always wanted. Write down your affirmations. Keep going back to these notes and read them to yourself every day. Write about your achievements so far. Make a list of things that are you're thankful for. Write about your previous day and what made you smile. Write about things you'd like to change and improve.

Journaling is having a conversation with your subconscious self, affirming your desires in an indirect manner. This ritual is a beautiful way to direct your frequencies towards ways & means to achieve your goals.

Nature

Nature has a very high vibration. By spending time outside and walking barefoot, we become part of a process called "Earthing". Earthing allows our bodies to receive a charge of beneficial energy fast. We used to all live in nature and were always synced with its energy & frequency.

With the industrial & technological developments we have gained a lot of good, but we have also lost a lot of good. With time we have completely lost touch with those vibrations, ultimately resulting in several problems like depression, anxiety, stress, etc. The syncing of our vibrations with 'Mother Earth' is extremely necessary for our wellbeing

It only makes sense that nature grounds us and surrounds us with positive energy. When surrounded by nature, our ego starts to dissolve, our low frequencies start to dissipate, and we raise our vibration. Spend time outside your home. Make an effort to sit in the sunlight and saturate yourself for at least 20 minutes a day to activate the good vibes inside you. Walk barefoot on grass or soil and notice how your energy changes. Go for a walk and notice the trees, the plants, and the birds. They are a part of us which we have all forgotten about. Sync yourself back to the frequency of earth and notice the positive changes inside you.

The ritual of spending time in nature, being close to plants, soaking the sunlight, breathing outside in open air daily will start transforming your body, mind & soul. Your stress level will go down considerably. Your mood will start staying positive. Your energy level will elevate and you will notice an overall improvement in your being.

Protection

This Universe is the most beautiful place yet it has some negative energy & entities in there as well. We are in constant struggle with these negative entities like our own dark side. Protection from these are also important for us. If we want to raise our vibration & elevate our frequency, we are in a consistent power struggle with the negative energies. They try to bring us down, they redirect our attention to take different decisions than the right ones, to deter us from our path.

The ritual of protection is very simple yet very powerful. It's all a game of energy & mind power. Use your sacred power of thought to imagine a white light beaming with love and protection. Imagine this sacred gleaming light surrounding you, your loved ones, and your home. This ritual adds a shield of protection from the dark side of this universe that we are in. This is a quantum reality and anything is possible. A simple sacred 'Protection Ritual' will repel any negative energy trying to enter your surroundings keeping you and your loved ones safe and secure and not hindering in your vibrations' ascension.

The Nourish Zone

Food is not a treat nor punishment. It's a sacred ritual by which you honor your temple (your body) and take care of its nourishment by providing the best nutritional choices. Commercial industry has programmed our minds to connect food with pleasure, treat, taste & cravings; which is the reason we have an obesity epidemic now. Our bodies are not made to eat the way the commercial industries have been promoting. Their reason is to make money whereas we are destroying our temples; our bodies.

Alter your perception about food being a source of treat, comfort or reward, think of food as fuel. Your body needs the right nutrients to work at its optimum level.

Nourishing our body is a sacred ritual just like breathing. When we provide our body with sun-drenched alive nutritious foods like plants, vegetables, fruits, seeds & nuts, we are technically preserving our treasure and enhancing its worth. Every bite we place in our mouth has a vibration; low or high. Imagine taking a bite of a crispy fresh summer salad drenched with micro and macro nutrients giving each cell of your body an ultimate boost and power.

"Every time you eat or drink, you are either feeding disease or fighting it."

—Heather Morgan

Honor your body; make a conscious effort to select the best food. Make grocery shopping a sacred ritual with time & effort to select the best for yourself. You cannot raise your vibration if all you are consuming is artificial, synthetic, and low vibrational food. Make a strong conscious effort to consume whole foods that mother earth gifts us every day drenched with its love and energy.

Not having time is just an excuse; it's all about priority and your desire to eat better. Take 1-2 hours every Sunday to prepare for the week and you will have the entire week of nourishing food every day. In the end, we really are what we eat. An abundance of positive energy, spiritual enhancement, emotional & mental clarity, and inner peace, all start with what we nourish our bodies with. Our food choices affect us on a mental, physical, emotional & spiritual level.

Food can simply be identified as dead or alive. Dead foods are cooked meats, dairy, processed food, junk food, etc. Dead food drains your energy and leave your body with a deficit of energy and health. Alive food is raw fruits and vegetables, nuts, seeds, and anything that is in its natural form. Alive foods are Gaia Food; blessed from mother earth. Gaia food gives you more energy than required for their digestion. A daily intake of such food selection provides you optimum energy level, enhances your mental clarity and focus, improves your emotional wellbeing, and most of all protects you from diseases. We are programmed to choose our meals based on taste. Change your perception and select foods based on their nutritional value and the health benefits they provide your body, mind, and soul. Always think of the consequence of your food selection not how it tastes. When you prepare your 'Gaia Meal'; always ask yourself, what benefit or consequence will I get for the food that I am selecting for my body?

Understanding the concept of higher vibration food is all about clear distinction between dead and alive food. 'Gaia Food' is drenched with sunlight, saturated with earth's love, and is perishable. The macronutrients and micronutrients found within these high vibrational foods are the secret. The energy, frequency & vibrational that these foods provide are more than physical. They are a direct source of enhancing our mental, emotional, and spiritual energy. Every single thing in this universe has its own energy, frequency & vibration and that includes food. Now imagine fueling your body, your temple with only the best high vibrational choices. Simply explained; eating low vibration food lowers your own vibration while eating high vibration food helps you elevate it.

Higher Vibration Foods

High vibration food is "Alive" food drenched with sunlight, earth energy & valuable nutrients containing a high vibration; they are natural and organic. They are not modified at any level. There is nothing added to them at all; you can find them locally especially at your farmers market. They are produced with no chemicals or additives.

A pure high vibrational ingredient is the one that is produced without chemicals, preservatives, or additives and gets its energy solely from either the sun, Earth, or natural water. So, anything that is not modified at any stage, is grown locally (Preferably) and naturally in its rawest form is a high vibrational food.

Instead of making things complicated; just make it a ritual to make your meals based on fruits, vegetables, herbs, seeds & nuts; natural, organic, and pure ingredients from the earth. You can find them locally at your farmers' market or you can also grow your own food which by experience I learnt is one of the easiest things to learn and manage even in smaller places. Avoid any food that is genetically modified as it messes with your system, No

GMOS, seedless, processed, persevered with chemicals, or canned. This ritual alone will have massive benefits to your nourishment ritual. Your body will naturally achieve its healthiest weight when you fuel it the right way. It will naturally eliminate unwanted fat, toxins & chemicals from itself once it's fueled right. Honor your body the way it was always meant to be.

This zone is about honoring your natural circadian cycle of consuming the right food at the right time to heal & nourish your mind, body & soul. 'Our Gaia', 'Mother Earth' gifts us miraculous, magnificent, powerful, valuable & nutritious foods every single day yet most of us go after processed & fast food destroying our body every day leading to diseases. We ignore these treasures and go after disease-laden junk.

Incorporate these treasures in your everyday meal plans and notice how your body, mind & soul starts upgrading. Your emotional state will improve. Select seasonal fruits & vegetables every day for your meals, add powerhouses like seeds; chia seeds, flax seeds, pumpkin seeds, sesame seeds, sunflower seeds, hemp seeds, etc. Flavor with an unlimited choice of natural herbs like basil, oregano, dill & natural grown supplements like turmeric, Himalayan salt, etc. Drizzle organic olive oil, grapeseed oil, or avocado oil on your meals. Enhance with jewels like cilantro, mint, etc. to add flavor. Use natural supplements like Matcha, Moringa, Ashwaghandha, Senna, etc. according to your body requirements. Understand the usage and benefits of these treasures to use them the right way for a well-balanced body. Hydrate your cells not only with water but water-based vegetables & fruits so your hydration is at cellular level not just topical.

There are many different nutritional researches and practices. There are unlimited books & diets. My belief is in balance, staying true to nature & cherishing earth's treasures. Gradual change and commitment are the secret.

The right time & the right way to fuel our body

Intermittent fasting reboots your entire system. It is the secret to valuable benefits like great skin and longevity. When you fast for 12-14 hours you maintain your health and when you fast for 16 hours plus a day you activate cleansing/fat-burning mode in your body. Keeping your eating window to 6-8 hours a day is optimum for health and longevity. It cleanses your body, super charges your organs and boosts weight loss immediately. Once you have achieved your desired weight loss you can resume back to the 12-14 hour fast. Once your body gets accustomed to the new routine it transitions to repair and rejuvenation mode daily.

When we restrict our eating window to certain hours, our body finally has time to do other important tasks like detoxifying & healing rather than constantly digesting food. The body automatically gets into a fat-burning/ cleansing mode rather than in constant digestion mode. Every organ has its own function to do at its specific timings. When we are constantly eating, we are depriving the body to function at its optimum level.

Cleansing & detoxifying is a major ritual performed by our body which is neglected tremendously when we are constantly feeding; forcing it to continuously digest food. When eating occurs at random times throughout the day and night, the body is constantly in the digestion mode and when you are disciplined in a routine of specific eating hours and timings with nutritious selections of food, your body turns into a self-healing, fat-burning machine. By conforming to sporadic eating timings, you throw your body out of sync and into constant pressure. Timing is vital and what you chose to eat is equally critical for your health.

Eating at the same time every day is one of the most powerful ways to keep your body in sync with your circadian rhythm. When we eat randomly throughout the day, our body has to keep insulin production active constantly, which directs our organs to keep making body fat. Having a defined eating time and duration also revives our hormone production and places it back to its natural rhythm as per our body's need. Surprisingly you will have more energy when you are not eating too much infact the brain works better on an empty stomach.

When you restrict your timings of consuming food, it reduces the pressure on your body to store more fat, and infact restores your body's own rhythm to heal and burn unnecessary fat. Your body cells and organs need several hours of rest and fasting at night to turn on their fat-burning mechanism hence your constant eating deprives you of this natural fantastic feature. This restriction reduces the body's drive to make or store excess fat, activates fat burning systems, normalizes cholesterol, improves blood pressure, and reduces inflammation in your body. Most importantly after several weeks of being on intermittent fasting, time-restricted eating, and the circadian rhythm, the nervous system activates as well helping your brain to heal and function at optimum levels.

Hence, Restriction on eating timings not only promotes weight loss, it's a beautiful ritual to help restore your health and activate your body's natural circadian rhythm for optimum performance and generates natural disease fighting mechanism.

I have personally incorporated Intermittent Fasting in my life and I am thrilled at the results. I have more energy than ever. My cravings have disappeared and I'm more emotionally stable. I lost all the extra weight I wanted to lose within 12 weeks.

Intermittent Fasting benefits may include:

- Reduction in body weight
- Increase in muscle mass
- Improved heart health
- Helps in normalized blood pressure
- Lower risk of type 2 diabetes
- Improved brain health
- 'Human Growth Hormone' increase
- Induction of cellular repair
- Reduced risk of diseases like cancer
- Reduced levels of inflammation in body
- Helps in normalized glucose levels
- Helps in normalized cholesterol levels
- Improved sleep quality
- Improved level of energy
- Helps prevent Alzheimer's disease
- Healthy gut
- Regular bowel movement
- Healthy kidney & liver function
- Helps longevity

Results vary depending on your other lifestyle choices and your current disease levels

Autophagy

The word 'autophagy' is derived from Greek words "auto" meaning self and "phagy" meaning eating. Autophagy literally means self-eating. It is a normal physiological ritual of the body that cleanses out damaged cells. Restricted timings of eating/intermittent fasting is known to activate autophagy. It is the process by which the body goes in the mode of eating out/cleansing all damaged cells. This mechanism provides fuel for the body and cleanses out all damaged cells hence regenerating the entire system activating new healthy cells. Our body is meant to heal itself in all circumstances & constantly improve its state; only if we give it the free time to perform the healing activates. Give it a break from constant eating & digesting, give it nutritious Gaia food in a restricted time span daily and watch your body's optimum state return.

Physical Zone

Exercise is a celebration of what your body can do; not a punishment for what you ate."

—Anonymous

Exercise literally relaxes the brain, reduces depression and anxiety, increasing our ability to experience happiness and tranquility. Incorporating exercise with intermittent fasting or restricted time of eating will literally melt away any unnecessary and unhealthy fat from your body; activating healing. Every morning jump-start your body by performing any physical activity of your choice such as stretching, walking, running, yoga, Tai-Chi, dancing, jumping jacks, planks, cycling, trampoline, swimming, sun salutations, Qi-Gong, Tibetan rites or home workout videos.

We thrive as humans if we nourish our body the right way and continue constant physical activity. If we don't; our bodies start to wilt. It's a natural response to not being in its natural state. Physical activity significantly enhances our health, keeps our emotions in a balanced state, providing health & longevity. Our energy levels depend on the amount of physical activity we choose every day. Activity can be anything that makes our body move, increases our heart rate, and gets our blood pumping and flowing in all parts of our body filling our lungs with pure oxygen, activating every cell in our body, and bringing it to life.

We can exercise any time of the day but if we activate your body in the morning it will provide us with life-long benefits. Even if it's just 10-20 min every morning, the results are remarkable.

Our body's lymphatic system is unable to flow on its own. It completely relies on us to move our body throughout the day in order for it to transport nutrients to our cells and detoxify them at the same time removing waste. The lymphatic fluid can start flowing with any kind of physical movement that our body experiences. It can start flowing with deep breathing, walking, taking the stairs, stretching; any movement that we initiate for our body will activate this system, and circulation of our lymphatic fluid will start. Lack of physical activity ages the cells in your body at a faster rate.

The goal is to activate our body and trigger its peak performance state by moving all fluids inside the right way. Exercise is a celebration of our physical activity level and stamina. It is indeed a blessing if we conceive exercise as a gift. Don't think of exercising as going to a gym and lifting weight or running on a treadmill. Exercise is the natural ritual that keeps our body at its functionality peak. Exercise is not to be hated but cherished. Incorporate physical activity in your day at all moments that you can by riding a cycle instead of taking the car, by walking instead of driving to nearby places, by swimming to relax, by taking stairs rather than the elevator or the escalator, by taking a stroll during lunch hour, by enjoying the trail on weekends instead of I Hop, by kayaking on a Sunday rather than sleeping in, by hiking on a Sunday afternoon rather than late night clubbing. Create a lifestyle where you choose to add movement every single day of your life in many different moments. Choose to be active rather than sedentary. This ritual of movement for your body will benefit your body to the extreme. This is the best gift you can give to yourself. Human body is made to be physically active.

Your morning activation exercise doesn't need to replace your afternoon running, gym, or workouts. Those have their own benefits. The more physical activity you incorporate in your life, the better your quality of life will be. Incorporating a few minutes of morning exercise ritual will have miraculous benefits on your health as it aids in healing blood sugar levels, blood pressure, heart health, osteoporosis, cancer, diabetes, and more. It activates your body at the start of the day providing you benefits throughout the day and years to come with consistent schedule. Physical activity not only energizes and heals your body, it brings power to your mind. Exercise has a very strong correlation with the mind. Your brain performance is enhanced and multiplied with regular exercise.

I usually like to go for a walk in the morning listening to motivational podcasts. This starts my day with a positive mindset, activates my body, and gets my blood pumping. After that, I take a shower and go in my quiet space for my meditation rituals. I have personally experienced continuous positive results with my rituals in the morning. Morning physical activity benefits include exposure to daylight which reduces depression and increases alertness. You naturally raise your level of cortisol to a healthy level which lowers inflammation.

Incorporate four kinds of physical activities in your life to keep the body strong, balanced, active, and vigorous. Exercises that

1. Boost the cardiovascular system. For example, walking, cycling, swimming, hiking, etc.

2. Create Strength. For example, weight training & body weight exercises.

3. Create Flexibility. For example, stretching.

4. Provide Balance. For example, yoga, tai chi, etc.

Learning Zone

Learning is the acquisition of knowledge to improve ourselves. We as humans have two choices, to grow or perish. This zone incorporates rituals you can select to improve, upgrade, and enhance yourself. There are numerous rituals in this zone that you can select from to meliorate yourself every single day. With all the technological advancements, information is at your fingertips every moment. It's your choice what you prioritize and focus on.

We all have 24 hours in a day, it's how we utilize those hours that define our life and success. We spend hours browsing on social media yet we don't spend 60minutes on an informational podcast or reading every day. There are unlimited streams of learning around us yet we chose to waste our time, attention & energy on mindless social media browsing.

We need to start using social media more intentionally, based on learning, educating & improving ourselves.

You can follow people who motivate and inspire you. Engage and learn from experts in your field of interests, spend time on learning new skills, let positivity and inspiration appear on your pages instead of negativity or low vibration materials.

The 'Learning Zone' is a very vital combination of rituals to elevate our mind & soul. You can select from reading, podcasts, seminars, workshops, or any source that helps you absorb new and quality information every single day. Learn new information, a new skill, or a new perspective; learn & constantly improve yourself. Challenge your mind constantly.

The greatest minds in human history have spent years acquiring knowledge and then transferring that knowledge in the form of books for people to read, learn, and take advantage from them. Books are treasures; words are information condensed from intellectual minds & experiences teaching us to learn and apply this treasure of knowledge to achieve the same level of success or more.

In my experience when you read a book you absorb the information according to the level of evolution that you are at. I have read the beautiful book "Alchemist" by Paulo Coelho three times in the past decade and every time it gives me more information and value than the last. You can choose any form of learning that resonates with your soul. If you are more of an audio learning person, you will sync best with an audio learning opportunity every day. Choose what's best for you but do this ritual every single day and improve yourself dramatically over the years of your life.

The Learning Zone is a silent elevation of your mind & soul.

It slowly and surely takes you on the path of enlightenment resulting in raising your vibration and ultimately attracting success and achievements your way. What you choose to learn is based on your interests and when you enhance your knowledge in your fields of interest, you raise your vibration accordingly. Having the desire to learn is a treasure.

"I'm still learning".

—Michelangelo (at age 87)

This zone focuses on investing in yourself and upgrading yourself constantly. Surround yourself with rituals that improve you constantly. Surround yourself with people who are smarter than you, who are learned and determined. Keep yourself around evolved, intelligent, successful people. If you are the smartest person in your circle you need to upgrade your circle. Be in a constant zone of learning and improving. Invest and join in groups and activities yielding high growth and wisdom. Build your network around such people. Your net worth is directly proportional to your network.

"You are the average of the five people you spend most of your time with."

—Jim Rohn

Creative Zone

What you are doing every single day is exactly what you are becoming. Where you are now is a direct result of how you have spent your days in the past few years. Maintaining an active mind is one of the key factors in staying young. Presented with new information and creativity is revitalizing to your mind. It's of utmost importance to expose yourself to creative avenues and to change. Challenging the brain makes it work at a higher level. Indulge yourself daily in at least one activity that enhances your creative aura. This ritual will benefit you in enormous ways mentally and emotionally.

We are literally wired to follow a mechanical schedule of work and we have forgotten to stop and smell the roses. This zone encourages you to explore your creative side and incorporate activities that you love in your everyday routine. These activities will give you power over your day.

"The best use of imagination is creativity."

—Deepak Chopra

Analyze yourself since your childhood and make a list of creative activities that you enjoyed doing. You can honor your creative side by assigning 30 minutes to an hour in your daily routine to your creative hobbies. These rituals collectively enhance your mind, body & soul;

elevating your vibrational level since you are making a conscious effort to improve yourself.

Explore your creative side and select activities that make you forget everything and be in the moment. These can be activities like painting, writing, gardening, embroidery, knitting, chess, crafts, dancing, flower arrangements, jewelry making, sewing, singing, playing instruments, etc. The list is endless when you explore your inner creative aura.

This zone enhances your own self as you spend time creating your own little treasures. There is immense satisfaction in watching things come together with your own creativity.

Prosperity Zone

Most of us have this preconceived notion that we are successful when we have a lot of money. The fact is that money is a by-product of success. Strive for excellence and be of service; abundance will follow. Don't be worried about numbers and money, be of service, and benefit to humanity. Prosperity & wealth is based on a beautiful law of nature which is the "Equation of Mutual Exchange". When you create and contribute towards the benefit of humanity and towards their service and prosperity, only then you will prosper in return and sustain that wealth & abundance for your entire life on this earth. Pure intentions, service, and prosperity of fellow humans, creation, and benefit to others create prosperity for you in return. It's a powerful phenomenon.

"Success is not the result of making money. Earning money is the result of success and success is in direct proportion to our service."

—Earl Nightingale

Our current situation, circumstances, and financial conditions are simply equivalent to our thoughts, Intentions, and level of benefit or service to humanity.

Prioritize & Focus

The real superpower behind all successful people is 'FOCUS'. Laser focusing on the right things with a master mindset instead of doing everything with a mediocre mindset is the key to achievement. Focus your attention on the activities that create self-discipline for you and that create future results for you. Identify and engage in activities that yield results instead of stagnancy. You don't need to be busy; you need to work smarter and focus your time and energy on the 'RIGHT' things. Attain clarity of your situation, identify the highest priority tasks, and laser-focus your energy towards them. There is a difference in being busy and being productive. Concentrate all your energy towards productive tasks to yield successful results.

"The successful warrior is the average man, with laser-like focus."

—Bruce Lee

For an uninterrupted day and to keep my focus on important tasks I keep my phone on silent all day. This avoids any unnecessary distractions that may consume my time and waste my precious moments. This silent ritual of my phone blocks any calls, emails, messages, or notification sounds that may trigger my attention towards it with every single bell. My phone is on silence mode since 2011. This is a simple ritual that dramatically increased my daily productivity and my ability to remain focused on the tasks in front of me. Designate a time during the day when you return all phone calls or messages as per your schedule. (Obviously, this works best if you are in a work/home situation where you can handle your phone being in silent mode). You can have certain notifications for any emergencies with family and friends etc. realistically unless you are an emergency room physician, you don't need to be instantly accessible to everyone. You can take your time to respond. There were times we all lived without phones and survived. This ritual will ease your dependency on the phone, will reduce the constant habit of checking your phone and being a slave to every notification.

For focus and results make a list of daily tasks that you do and analyze what can be taken off as unnecessary and time-wasting. Review your list over and over again and analyze which tasks can be delegated, deleted, or automated. Prioritize tasks according to their importance to you. Spend most of your time on tasks that produce results in your life.

Arigato Your Money

The Japanese Entrepreneur Wahei Takeda's Success Mantra

Money is more or less a necessity to survive in this world but many of us have associated money with a negative emotion with either fear or hate. Money is not a negative entity; it can be seen bringing us joy, gratitude, and happiness, especially when we give it away as charity with a free heart and with the same positive energy as we receive it.

We see money as lifeless paper. How about interacting with your money. Giving it value (not greed, fear, or hate); in fact, positive abundant importance & respect. There are several ways to create a happy flow of money, including donating to a charity, giving to friends & family in need, and gifts. There are a few more interesting ways to interact with your money in a way that will make your relationship to your finances more positive. Always remember to never fall in the trap of greed, jealousy, comparison, fear, hate, or stinginess regarding money.

Arigato means 'Thank you'; a magical word. 'Thank you', 'Merci', 'Shukran', 'Grazie', 'Gracias', 'Tesekkur', 'Alhamdolillah'; they are absolutely extraordinary words. Gratitude is in itself a phenomenal ritual.

"The most profound lesson in making and securing good fortune came to me from Wahei Takeda, my mentor. He once told me a story of a man who came to him in desperation. The man had massive amounts of debt and needed money. Wahei said he would give him the money but only if he said arigato (thank you) 100,000 times. That meant he would have to say arigato every minute

of the day for months on end. The man agreed. By the time he went to borrow money, he no longer needed it. Why? His mindset of appreciation started to reap its own rewards. He was able to pay off his debts and no longer needed to borrow the money. When we say thank you, we release powerful energy into the world. We are instantly present. We realize everything we have is enough. We are enough. We have all that we need. Knowing this and feeling this is the most powerful force in the universe. You can literally achieve anything when you ground yourself in appreciation and gratitude."

—Ken Honda

The Extra Mile

Always go the 'Extra Mile' for anything and anyone. Giving extra than expected in any deal, business, transaction or situation transforms the fearful, awkward, reluctant, doubting, and anxious energy into a positive force that leaves people feeling like they are appreciated and valued. It is almost like taking a step of an investment in the emotional health, well-being, and treasure of your own being and souls around you.

When you exceed any expectations, you stand out immediately. Even if you are not appreciated for the effort, your spiritual elevation takes place. It's a superb way to raise your vibrations every day and to create a positive relationship with money.

The Secret Mantra

Leave people with more than they have given you and you'll be automatically on the universe's receiving side. It's almost a selfish yet selfless ritual. Leave people with more than they expect. If someone gives you something, always give more in return and you will be a magnet for abundance as you become a medium to 'GIVE' more than others. When you are always in the 'Giver' state you are chosen by the universe over others as you have the selfless heart to freely help & give.

Remain on the giving end of the universe's givers & receiver's chain and you will have endless abundance. Detach yourself from money but value it immensely. Give freely as much as possible to stay in the 'GIVER's' zone.

When someone gives you something, they are in the 'Giver's Zone' and you are in the 'Receivers Zone'. Change the dynamic right away and return them eventually with more than they gave you and you alter your zone immediately entering the 'Giver's mode'. This is the zone of abundance; the secret Mantra.

Giving: A Beautiful Ritual

Giving is an extraordinary law in the universe that gives you peace and multiplies your funds enormously, taking you on the track of abundance in massive ascension. Once you commit to the ritual of giving in your life, you elevate yourself at a frequency that will attract receiving at a magnificent pace.

Giving can be anything; money, your time, physical things like food, clothes, medicines, etc. The ritual of being in the zone to always willingly give to others creates a magnet attraction of receiving from the universe in your aura.

When you commit yourself to be constantly in the 'Givers Mode'; you sync with the Universe's attribute and the universe returns your ritual in multiples. This simple law of universe; the law of giving, elevates you to the frequency of abundance.

Prosperity Synopsis in the world dimension

1.   First and foremost, *secure your monthly income* that pays your bills and always give it the time and attention it needs as this is your financial base for now. Honor this source as this will give you the foundation to go out and generate more sources.

2.   *Evaluate your unique skills, traits, and strengths.* Every soul on earth has his own exclusive and individual skills that are like no other that can generate compensation in return. Any skill that you have that may offer value to others can generate an income source for you. Analyze your knowledge, ability, education, skill, or experience that may add value to others. You are unique and there is no one else like you. Identify things that you are good at and things that you love doing. List them out and analyze how you can create an income source out of them.

3.   *Increasing your knowledge* in varied areas of interest to you will enhance your abilities further and become an income source for you eventually. Take an hour a day for reading, listening to podcasts, or enrolling in online programs or workshops to enhance your knowledge.

4.   *Determine your target audience*; the people who can benefit exclusively from the knowledge and skills that you have. What can you do to make their lives better? What is the problem for them that you can solve? What is the way you can enhance their lives? What value can you add to their lives?

5.   Classify your audience based on different knowledge, traits, and skills that you have and create solutions or value information accordingly. Now take this one step at a time and put all your energy into the *first source* that you have identified.

Organize the necessary steps needed to initiate and launch that source. It could be your passive income source or active source depending on which quality you have identified and how you will create the source. And in the same way slowly and surely take all your attributes and start generating income sources for yourself resulting in financial freedom in your future.

6.   There are many other opportunities to add to your passive income sources and these include rental income, property appreciation, investments in stocks and bonds, etc. The most important ritual is to make sure you isolate one hour every week to analyze and organize your income streams. This is the path to financial abundance and savings and the right investments for yield is the path to financial freedom.

7.   Organize your life and create systems. This is an extremely valuable step towards security and abundance. Generating systems will free your time to focus on the more important stuff rather than wasting your time and energy on less important tasks. Organize your life, your day, and create systems in every place that you can so that you are free to engage in more valuable activities resulting in improving yourself and success.

8.   You have technically four resources in your life; your mind, money, people, and time. Use these sources very wisely. Spend

each one of those wisely to get the greatest return. You are a genius elevating your financial stature; train yourself to delegate 80% of the work and keep the vital 20% for yourself.

9. Create accountability for yourself. Be smart in making money and be smarter in saving/investing money and be extremely smart in where you are spending money.

Passive income sources

Learn how to create passive income sources so you don't have to depend on one. Earning money is not an issue, learning how to save money and multiplying it is the art we need to learn. Always set aside 10% of your income to save and invest. Take 10% of your income and give it to charity. This is the best formula for success; 'Giving'. You have to teach your subconscious mind that there is abundance surrounding you and by giving you attract ten times more. Holding on makes it stale and you stop the cycle of abundance. There is enough for everyone and more. You just need to have faith and tap into it and you will have unlimited resources flowing to you.

Platinum Prosperity Hour

Schedule a time every weekend, an hour where you just brainstorm, identify, analyze, and initiate your passive or active income sources.

This ritual is extremely vital for your financial security and growth. We are so used to the weekly work, sleep, eat routine that we forget to think outside of it. Halt your weekly routine and every Sunday morning give yourself one hour for your future and your financial freedom. This hour will generate your passive income source ideas and give you hope & growth. Analyze your strengths, skills, and talents and write down the multiple ways that you can generate passive income sources. You just need a positive mindset and faith to coordinate and initiate these sources and one by one they will start yielding results. Make this a priority in your life. Identify your talents and income streams ideas and diversify them in different areas so you are safe. Identify and create passive & active income source.

Recovery Zone

In spirituality, the concept of sleeping is for your conscious mind to rest, while your spiritual being is attuned to your higher realm syncing with the natural laws of the universe attaining experiences & wisdom necessary to advance. Technically speaking when your body is resting, your conscious mind is in off-mode but your soul is at the highest vibration charging, aligning, syncing, reminiscing itself with the infinitely magical frequency of the universe.

Our modern lifestyle is disrupting our primitive system; the 'Circadian Rhythm" of our body. Circadian rhythms are the biological rituals and processes that every living thing experiences throughout the 24 hours. It aligns and activates our systems with sunrise and sunset. Our ancestors followed the circadian rhythm and naturally experienced strength, vitality, and happiness. Restoring to our natural rhythm of living and syncing back to our rituals will result in the resolution of our health mentally & physically. The human body is designed to follow the natural cycle for optimum health. When we disrupt the rhythm, we initiate and activate all health issues like the ones we experience today. Anxiety, depression, ADHD, Insomnia, obesity, diabetes, dementia, cardiovascular diseases, blood pressure, infections, migraines, and even many serious diseases like cancer, etc. These are all more or less the result of our lifestyle.

The good news is that you can re-boot your system and sync yourself back to the rhythm that the universe has scheduled for your body to take care of it properly.

Our body is a complex system and it works like a miracle performing all that it does internally. Every organ in our body goes through a very specific ritual of healing and working operating at specific times performing vital tasks. Circadian rhythm simply guides us when to eat and when to turn off the lights. It directs us to the right timing to nourish our body and rest to recover and rejuvenate properly. Resting and repairing is the most vital ritual for our body. The right timings for it assimilate the optimum levels. Rest is the healing time for our body. At night the brain detoxifies and heals. All toxins are cleaned up when we sleep and new brain cells are developed through the process of neurogenesis. Intermittent fasting also enhances the process of neurogenesis.

Our physiology is pretty much the same as it was millions of years ago. We are meant to sleep at night and work/eat during the daytime. Our internal clocks are synced with sunrise and sunsets naturally. This is the programming of our internal clock which stays the same no matter how much we evolve. This basic rhythm needs to be followed in order to sustain ourselves to optimum levels of health & vitality.

The natural circadian rhythm incorporates rising with the sun and resting when the sunsets. The early morning hours of the day are the best hours to be utilized for soul elevation and starting your work. The hours after sunset are meant for relaxation and rest and should be spent accordingly. These days the artificial lights and the bright screens disrupt our circadian rhythms, reduce our sleep hormone melatonin keeping us awake hence affecting our natural rhythm. Low exposure to sunlight or daylight affects our proper alignment with the natural rhythm. These habits result in insomnia, depression, anxiety, migraine, irritation, mood swings, ADHD, and many other disorders and onset of diseases.

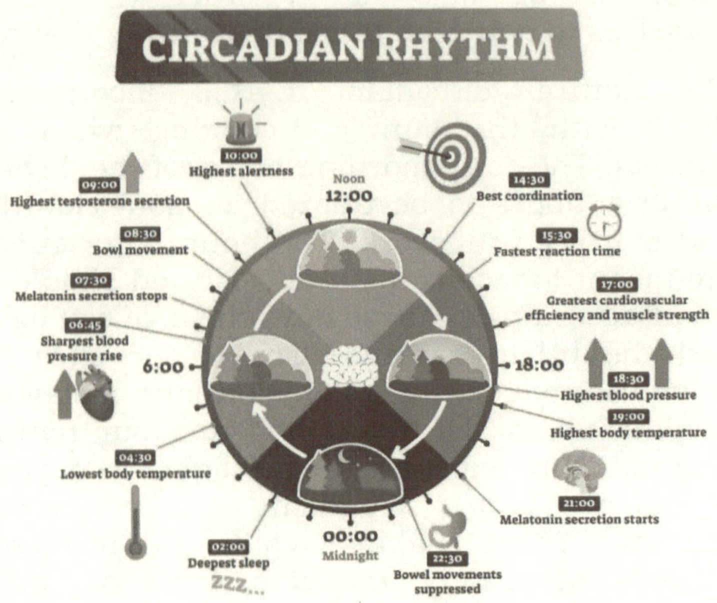

The best way to reset our circadian rhythm is by disciplining our evening routine. Once we establish a healthy significant evening schedule incorporating the 7 zones discussed in this book with highlighting the golden hour of the evening, we will automatically reset our rhythm and sync back to our original default settings. We live in a world now which is activated 24/7. There is no difference between day and night. Our news channels, entertainment channels, social media, everything is working and available 24/7. It's unbelievably hard to detach from this and discipline ourselves. Yet taking that decision will be the single most important step we will take towards our own betterment.

The virtual world is at our fingertips without disruption. The entire world is available to us with a single click any time of the day or night hence making us addicted. This lifestyle has completely disrupted our natural circadian cycle throwing us completely off sync hence we are suffering from all sorts of diseases and issues physically and mentally like obesity, depression, anxiety, sadness, low energy, etc.

Sleep

Sleeping is one of the most vital parts of our day. It recovers our body from the day's activity and prepares our body for the next day's energy. Sleep restores, rejuvenates, and recovers our mind, body, and soul. It gives us longevity, aids in lowering stress levels and provides our body eight hours of nonstop cleansing, detoxifying, and rejuvenation. Sleep is a very vital anti-aging tool. Our body generates melatonin when we sleep. Melatonin is a very powerful antioxidant that strengthens the immune system, promotes the natural production of insulin, prevents osteoporosis, and protects against many diseases. Melatonin is a key ingredient in the body for preserving youth; hence your own secret fountain of youth.

Sleep timings every day are crucial for your body's health. Commit to your self –discipline ritual by having the same and regular sleep hours every single day. Be consistent in your routine. Try to change your habit of being on your phone the first hour after waking up and the hour before sleeping. Being on the phone dealing with the artificial light a few hours before bedtime is enough to throw you off sync, suppress your melatonin levels and disturb your sleep.

Rest (during the day)

We have pre-conceived notions that success only comes if we are busy all day. That is such a wrong approach. The idea is to work smarter not harder, create systems, and develop self-discipline in our daily rituals and selections. Another very important ritual is to rest. Resting doesn't have any scheduled time frame or reason. Your body is the best guide. Whenever you feel overwhelmed, exhausted, or tired, take a few moments in a quiet place to 'REST', close your eyes and take a power nap or just be in that calm quiet place in silence to recover. This ritual rejuvenates you and throws you back at your optimum levels to take charge of your day again. Instead of constantly being on the go, take a few short periods throughout the day as needed to enjoy silence, quiet time, sacred space, and restoring your energy levels.

The ritual of rest melts away stress and reboots your system powerfully. It helps lower your heart rate and blood pressure. Slowing down and easing yourself out of pressure helps you to hear your inner wisdom and knowledge that guides you best to handle everything. Resting allows peace, contentment, and relaxation into your life, healing you from inside out. Take short moments of rest throughout your day as needed and also take an entire day or weekend of rest as required. This ritual reboots your system resulting in more energy levels than before.

Insomnia

I, personally, have suffered from the terrible experience of insomnia for years after the incident that changed my life. I could not sleep and whenever I slept, I would keep waking up multiple times throughout the night staring at the ceiling, getting up very tired the next day. Insomnia is truly painful experience for those who suffer from it. In my quest to find solutions to my sufferings, I tried many different rituals to ease myself through sleepless nights.

Deep breathing, calming music, lavender oil aromatherapy, and my sleep meditation helped me conquer my insomnia to a great extent.

This sleep meditation is a ritual every night that ends my day in a tranquil manner taking me slowly to a very relaxed physical and mental state. My 'Evening Ritual' before sleeping constitutes:

- Lowered lights
- Comfortable attire
- Light relaxing music
- Quick planning & overview of my next day
- Prioritizing tasks for the next day
- No phone (at least an hour before sleep)
- Reading
- Gratitude minute
- Setting intentions for future goals & dreams
- Talking & activating my subconscious mind for solutions and guidance for the next day & the journey of my goals.
- Evening meditation

When you open your eyes the next morning, 'SMILE' and thank the universe for another beautiful day. Set the intentions for this day with gratitude, visualizations, affirmations, and by guiding your subconscious mind to exactly what you'd like to achieve.

Sleep Meditation Ritual

"I'm blessed to have another day in my life to co-create my reality. I'm ready to end my day and rest my mind & body to attain strength & vitality for the new day tomorrow. A beautiful sense of calmness surrounds me, feeling of tranquility encompasses my entire aura and every cell in my body is looking forward to my body resting and rejuvenating itself. This sleep is a blessing and it helps my body rest, detox, rejuvenate, recover & retain.

I feel my body relaxing and entering a healing, restful & serene state. Every part of my body from my toes to my crown chakra is relaxed. I feel the Divine Energy flow through me peacefully with love caressing every cell in my body to relax. My Infinite Source cradles me with love and surrounds me with protection. All through this night, I'll be loved, safe and protected.

I will wake up to a beautiful morning and another blessed day filled with the guidance and love of my Divine Power. I allow my Source Energy, my infinite Intelligence to guide me in all my worldly events & experiences and lead me towards all that I desire revealing all that is beneficial for my life path.

My Eternal Source Energy is flowing through me and I am going to experience the most beautiful, restful, serene sleep ever."

The 7 Zones; Daily Ritual Examples

Since I run my own business and work from home mostly, my schedule is flexible and I can break my zones in parts as it fits in my day. Also, I can't stay focused for too long at one thing so the best way for me is short increments of incorporating different zones. The goal is to make sure all zones are nourished in one day and I achieve that blissfully with my schedule as I know the importance of each

6:30 am – 9 am	*Soul Zone – Part 1* *Physical Zone – Part 1* *Learning Zone – Part 1*	Prayer | Meditation | Gratitude | Affirmations | Visualization 20-minute walk Podcast, videos, audio books with walk Shower, getting ready
9 am – 10 am	*Creative Zone*	60 minutes of writing
10 am – 11 am	*Prosperity Zone – Part 1*	Work tasks
11 am – 11:30 am	*Nourish Zone – Part 1*	First meal following intermittent fasting Nourishing breakfast
11:30 am – 3 pm	*Prosperity Zone – Part 2*	Work tasks
3:30 pm – 4:30 pm	*Physical Zone – Part 1*	Gym
4:30 pm – 7:30 pm	*Nourish Zone – Part 2*	Cooking dinner. Last meal of the day ends at 6:30 pm (family time/activities)
7:30 pm – 8:30 pm	*Prosperity Zone – Part 3*	Work tasks
8:30 pm – 9:30 pm	*Learning Zone -Part 2*	60 minutes of reading
9:30 pm – 10:30 pm	*Family Time*	:)
10:30 pm – 6:30 am	*Soul Zone – Part 2* *Recovery Zone*	Relaxation | Breathing | Gratitude | Affirmations | Visualization | Reprogamming subconscious mind 7 hours of blissful sleep

zone.

"Instead of saying 'I don't have time' try saying 'it's not a priority' and see how that feels. Often, that's a perfectly adequate explanation. I have time to do this, I just don't want to. Changing our language reminds us that time is a choice. We can choose differently."

—Wall Street Journal

Example of incorporating these zones with a 9-5 pm work schedule.

6 am – 8 am	*Soul Zone*	Prayer | Meditation | Gratitude | Affirmations | Visualization
	Physical Zone	30-minute walk or workout
	Learning Zone	Podcast, videos, audio books with walk Shower, getting ready
	Nourish Zone – Part 1	Nourishing breakfast
8 am – 9 am	*Family Time*	
9 am – 1 pm	*Prosperity Zone – Part 1*	Work tasks
1 pm – 1:30 pm	*Nourish Zone – Part 2*	Lunch
	Learning Zone – Part 2	Audio book, podcasts
1:30 pm – 5 pm	*Prosperity Zone – Part 2*	Work tasks
5 pm – 8 pm	*Family time*	Dinner
	Nourish Zone – Part 3	
8 pm – 9 pm	*Creative Zone*	Any activity that sparks creativity in you
9:30 pm – 10 pm	*Learning Zone – Part 3*	30 minutes of reading
10:30 pm – 6:30 am	*Soul Zone – Part 2*	Golden Hour Rituals
	Recovery Zone	7 hours of blissful sleep

Time is a mindset. You find time for things that you prioritize in life. It takes mindset, commitment, structure, faith, willpower & discipline to achieve. Think of your life in terms of an athlete's life. Every single second is important. Every single second of your life you can either grow or perish. Every single activity that you do determines whether you are growing or perishing.

You usually spend hours on your phone browsing. Going through mindless scrolling. What a waste of your own life. Change your habits. Prioritize every second of your day with powerful intense quality rituals that will ultimately define your life and take you towards achieving your goals.

Every day of your life, your body's powerful and magical immune system destroys a cell that would have become cancer if it had lived. Five major things that influence this phenomenon are:

1. Your thoughts!

2. What you nourish your body with; your food choices

3. What you breathe and how you breathe

4. Your physical activity level & choices

5. What your skin absorbs; your skincare choices & your environment

"Going after a dream has a price, it may mean abandoning our habits, it may make us go through hardships, or it may lead us to disappointment, but however costly it may be, it is never as high as the price paid by people who don't live it."

—Paulo Coelho

A personal note

My life is committed to healing souls & aligning people to their best-self, leading, and living a high vibrational lifestyle. I am sharing these life-changing rituals with you, guiding you to the best of my ability but in the end, you have to commit and follow these rituals so you can align your life to your purpose and live your life to the fullest potential that you have ever dreamt of. I can hold your hand and show you the direction but ultimately, it's your own commitment. Yes, it is all possible if you understand the importance behind these rituals and commit your heart and soul in following through. Resulting in your own life changing for the best that you could ever imagine.

Daily Rituals

- **Wake up with a smile**
  Conversation with your Source / Subconscious Mind / Reminder to glide through the day & life

- **Prayers**
  Positive Thoughts
  Love & Family
  Blessings

- **Meditation**
  Gratitude
  Affirmation
  Visualizations
  Deep Breathing

- **Learning**
  Podcasts
  Reading

- **Creativity**
  Writing, Painting, Gardening, or any creative ritual

- **Movement**
  Exercise
  Yoga
  Stretching
  Walk
  Nature/Sunshine

- **Nourishment**
  Plant-Based
  Superfoods
  Alive Food
  Alkaline diet

- **Prosperity**
  Productivity & Abundance
  Schedules

- **Evening**
  Reading
  Meditations
  Conversation with Source/Subconscious Mind
  Sleep peacefully

Part 4
The GAIA Diet

This nourishment ritual for your body is based on honoring 'The Gaia'; 'Mother Earth', trusting its treasures and philosophies, and nourishing every cell in your body with the perfectly nutritious ingredients that are naturally gifted to us from our 'Source Energy'; our universe.

The universe has blessed us with utmost treasures of naturally yielding food saturated with its love, energy, vibrations, nutrients & benefits. 'Mother Earth' knows what our body needs and it has nutrition in every single edible source for us to take advantage of. This is one of the best ways to raise your vibrations, by consuming high vibrational, alive food. Nourishing your body with the right ingredients in the right season at the right time is the key to attaining a healthy, energetic, optimally functioning body. The 'GAIA Diet' is a plant-based technique of alimentative plan that will heal your body and transform all its functions to the optimum level. It will help you manage your weight issues and prevent many diseases even before they can attack your system.

Behold, I have given you every plant yielding seeds that is on the surface of all the earth, and every tree which has fruit yielding seed; it shall be food for you." (Genesis 1:29)

The 'GAIA Diet' is based on the ancient way of nourishing our body. This is the methodology that was used by our ancestors. It's the vibrational essence of 'GAIA, 'Earth' to nurture every part of your body with the highest vibrational ingredients for it to function at its optimal level. It's based mainly on the authentic & natural sources of nutrition that 'The GAIA' gifts us to heal, nourish & transform our system. When you incorporate this methodology of food consumption, you will honor your mind, body, soul with the blessing of your 'Source Energy'.

Food is fuel, it's not comfort. Feeding your body is a mechanism to nourish it for it to perform its functions to the highest level possible. What you eat becomes you; you are what you eat. The system of food consumption that you have chosen in the last year, the last decade or all your life has resulted in the emotional & physical state that you are in right now. Your thoughts, your skin, your body weight, your emotions, your confidence, your activity level, your energy level, your aging scale and the overall state that you are in right now is 80% due to the choices of food that you have made in the past months & years. Our gut is deeply connected to our brain. Whatever we consume becomes us, becomes our thoughts, emotions, and our body.

"70% of your serotonin is made in your gut. What's going on in your gut is going to affect your mood- anxiety, depression & focus."

—Dr. Frank Lipman

We have to change our emotions with food. Our society has trained us to feed ourselves based on taste and emotions whereas the right manner to consume food is by its nutritive value to your body. Every meal should be planned based on the diversity and level of nutrition that it can provide your body instead of how it tastes.

Stop feeding your emotions, and start nourishing your body.

The wrong food choices disturb our entire frequency, lowers our vibrations, makes our body gain unnecessary fat, and invite all sorts of diseases. Our mental state is directly proportionate to our meal selections. Our energy level, emotional state, and overall balance is all dependent mainly on what we consume every day. Our body is our temple and we should be extremely protective about it. We are beautiful natural spiritual beings. Each one of us has a poetic unique body silhouette, beautiful in its own uniqueness, and we have covered it all up with unnecessary fat deposits due to severely bad food choices. Accept & honor your uniqueness, your individuality, your own aura but don't celebrate this unnecessary disease-laden fat on your body which invites diseases.

It's a result of the wrong food selections. Rise above this low vibrational system of feeding your temple and choose how you will nourish your body with the mindset of an owner of the temple.

Honor your body, value it, and cherish its functionalities.

Corporations today have programmed and paralyzed our minds. They have literally deformed our bodies into an unhealthy state just to make money for themselves and of us. 'Fast food', 'low fat', 'Canned', 'Processed', 'Seedless', 'Fat-free', 'Low calorie', etc. are just a few examples of their money-making empires. We are choosing ease, artificial taste, disease, and negativity for our bodies. We are constantly consuming and feeding our loved ones and family empty low vibrational calories.

A great example is; the calorie content of a large fast-food fries pack is approximately 510 Kcal. This is 510 Kcal of the worst quality of fat & carbohydrate that you can consume. Its 510 Kcal that are empty calories providing zero quality nutrition for your body. Whereas a large apple 'GAIA Inspired Food', has approximately 130 Kcal. This 130 Kcal are filled with quality nutrients, flavonoids, antioxidants, and dietary fiber. More importantly, the calories in an apple are termed as negative calories, which means that the body spends more energy digesting this food rather than the calories from the food turning into fat. Empty calories are deficient in nutrients and are the reason you accumulate fat on your body resulting in disease onset. This is the basic example of low vibrational food & high vibrational 'GAIA' inspired food.

Become a healthy, vibrant, glowing, high vibrational, optimum performing individual by making honorable choices for yourself. The 'GAIA Diet' is the epitome of non-extreme, nourishing choices that you can make in this modern world and achieve all the benefits.

The GAIA food choices are nutrient & antioxidant-rich and provide miraculous benefits. They are directly from mother earth, drenched with sun energy and without any alteration and modification; providing nutrients, micronutrients, vitamins, minerals, antioxidants, healing & quality nourishment.

The universe is 'Infinite Intelligence'; it is perfect wisdom. The food sources it provides for us encompasses high vibrations, value, meaning, healing, and natural nourishment that our body requires every day and each season. GAIA food choices provide us with a substantial amount of nutrients per calorie that we consume. GAIA is our power-diet, constructed to nurture all our significant organs with vitamins and nutrients that can help them thrive and function optimally.

Amber Khan

The Gaia Diet incorporates Fruits, Vegetables, Herbs, Nuts, Seeds, and Water. It is the simplest and most effective lifestyle to nourish your mind, body & soul through the treasures of Gaia.

The Two Golden Hours of Your Day

I used to always think that there is a formula out there that I need to find a scientific, mystical, or mathematical formula that is the key to happiness, serenity & success. The ultimate calculation which will help me lead my life to my goals and live the dream. After all these years of yearning, researching, thinking, calculating, studying, feeling, analyzing, and realizing, In the end, I finally figured out that formula. The magic formula is simply your daily rituals. How you live your day defines exactly how your life is going to be.

The simplicity of it blew me away.

Pay attention to your daily rituals especially the hour after you wake up and the hour before you sleep as they play a major role in programming your subconscious mind and ultimately anchors in defining your life and your path to success.

Think of these two hours as a goldmine and give it the utmost importance, attention, and care. You may have heard about some amazing books written on the importance of the morning hours like the miracle morning book series, the 5 am club, etc. They are all fabulous books and explain exactly what needs to be accomplished. There is a reason they all stress on the importance of these hours, they know the magic hidden in them. Avail the magic for your happiness and growth.

The Golden Hour of your Morning. (G.M)

As soon as you open your eyes from a restful sleep, your day starts. Every second after this counts to either your growth, stagnancy, or perishing. What would you choose out of the three? If you have this book in your hand it's a huge affirmation that you are on your way to healing and transformation. You are sick of everything that has not worked so far and you'd like to change, for the better. Welcome to the 1% of the population who is following these rituals and creating life exactly how they want it and enjoying peace, happiness, success, and growth.

How you start your day determines how the rest of your day will be and ultimately how your life will shape. The morning hour sets the tone and anchors your entire day. When you wake up in the morning, open your eyes and smile. Thank the universe for this beautiful new opportunity in your life; this new day. Start this day as if this is the last day of your life. Wake up with a purpose of living this day instead of dragging yourself through the hours. Your mindset at this hour will frame the rest of your 23 hours & eventually your life. Be happy, be excited, be optimistic, be energized, be thankful, and be full of positivity.

The first step after waking up is thanking the universe and talking to your subconscious mind. The same ritual that you will repeat in the evening. Keep your eyes closed and acknowledge its value and presence in your life. Talk about your goals and dreams and relay exactly how you want your day to go. Trust me it will give you directions & redirections beyond your wildest dreams. This is the simplest mechanism yet the most powerful one.

After waking up, have warm water with lemon and use the next 60 minutes for meditation, affirmations, visualizations, stretching & your morning workout or walk in nature. This is the soul zone of your day & these activities will reprogram your mind & transform your life into the best scenarios for you.

This 'Golden Hour' of your day will set the tone of your entire day. Use this magical time to its maximum benefit by incorporating these soul-satisfying rituals. These rituals will start raising your vibrations ultimately taking you to a state where you will start attracting your dreams and goals; your life will start transforming. Incorporate the 'Soul zone' rituals in Part 3 of this book to raise your vibration & align your soul to its purpose.

The Golden Hour of your Evening. (G.E.)

The hour before you sleep sets the tone of your 'Recovery zone' and ultimately is the base of your next new day. Your body and your conscious mind sleeps and rests but your subconscious mind is awake all those hours. Imagine what a miracle this is. You are asleep, but all your body functions are taking place guided by your subconscious mind. Your heart is beating, you are breathing, blood is pumping in all veins in your body, every cell is alive and working its scheduled tasks for the night, your body is healing and recovering in the most beautiful poetic rhythm of the universe's secret code, yet you are asleep. While this is your recovery zone, your subconscious mind is working 24/7, hence working throughout the night. The 60 minutes before you sleep are magical minutes to reprogram your subconscious mind to be the ultimate guide for your growth.

Use the golden hour of your evening to prepare for your recovery zone and assign tasks to your subconscious mind before you go to sleep so the hours that you are asleep, it's already working for your benefit. When you give it direction and specific words, it will work like a miracle for you.

"Never go to sleep without a request to your subconscious."

—Thomas A. Edison

Whatever you 'THINK' and 'FOCUS' on throughout your day is what your subconscious mind will absorb and ultimately guide you accordingly. If you are thinking sad thoughts, depressing memories, painful past all day, that's exactly what you will see throughout your day and dream through your night. You will come across depressing posts, sad news, negativity, low vibration souls in your average day, because your subconscious mind has been fed with a particular level of emotions all day, hence it will guide accordingly. But if you consciously make an effort to alter your thoughts to positivity; you will attract its frequency and start elevating your vibration. When you follow the rituals in this book, your entire system will start reprogramming itself, guiding you to the best things for your growth and success.

Evening Ritual

This is the winding down hour for you. Start preparations for your sleep. By this time try to finish up all your daily home & family rituals so this time is yours to cherish. Take a shower if you'd like, wear comfortable nightwear, lower the lights in your home and especially in your bedroom. Candlelight is beautiful at this time as it sets the tone for the night. Have beautiful calming relaxing music in your room.

By this moment you should be in a relaxed zone. You are done with your day. It's the last few minutes before you will close your eyes and sleep to rest and rejuvenate for the next new beautiful day. Sit on your bed in a comfortable position. Take some lavender oil and inhale a few times. This helps your frequency like magic. Take these few minutes and breathe deeply. 3-5-7. Breathe through your nose on the count of 3, hold for count of 5 and release through your mouth on count of 7. Repeat those a few times. This ritual will further take you in a very serene state of relaxation.

After this blow off your candle and lay down in your bed, get comfortable, now the most important minutes of this golden hour. Close your eyes and focus on your relaxed state of mind and body. Express gratitude for the day and your life, recite a few affirmations you love (short and concise). Lastly and most importantly, acknowledge and thank your subconscious mind. Think of your subconscious mind as a separate entity in your body and talk to it like a friend. At this moment think of anything that you'd like help within your life, any task that you'd like to be guided with, and deliver a request to it and then acknowledge it again and prepare yourself to sleep.

At this moment onwards something miraculous happens. You sleep but your subconscious mind actively processes your request and prepares to guide you in the best way possible. In the days and nights that you keep practicing this ritual, your life will start changing as your subconscious mind will start showing you exactly what you need to see during the day for your growth leading you to your dreams; you attract what you think.

The amount of information that you see on an average day is enormous but there is only so much that you can focus on and pay attention to. If you are constantly focusing on sad events in your thoughts or a painful past, you will notice that all you attract and see is sadness, negativity, and depressing things. But if you focus on being happy and all the good things in life, you will notice that you will start attracting similar frequencies. Your brain stores your emotions and then matches you with the same frequency information or events.

Since you are programming your subconscious mind every morning and evening to help you with your goals and dreams, it will start diverting your attention towards information and events relating to that. It's a miraculous magnetic formula.

Your Kingdom; Your Home

Cleanse Your Physical space for new energy

Your environment becomes you; you become what you surround yourself with. Energies are contagious; choose carefully. Transformation, evolvement, improvement, learning, spiritual elevation & the path to healing requires inside & outside work. You have to work with your heart, mind, soul, your physical body & your physical space. These are all interlinked & interconnected; hence physical space around us is equally important for our journey. We become what we are surrounded with, we become our environment.

Our physical space is our kingdom. We live here every single day; we breathe in its aura & air. Our kingdom is not only our defined physical space, our home, it's also who we surround ourselves with. You eventually become the five closest people to you. Think about this and reflect on its importance.

Physical environment mirrors our internal state. We can transform all we want inside but if our physical space is cluttered, dirty, unorganized & filled with stagnant dead energy, our journey will halt at one point. A disorganized and cluttered environment is stagnant negative energy and if this energy is not cleansed and turned into flowing positive vibrant energy, it will deteriorate us immensely directly or indirectly. Create room for fresh & better energy.

Personal physical space is mainly our home, our work area, and our mode of transport. De-clutter, organize, cleanse, disinfect, and minimalize; elevate the vibrational energy of your home. Keep this as your Sunday ritual to go through your home & car to remove any stagnant energy and refresh your surroundings.

If you look around your home, your closets, your drawers, your garage, your storage area; you will notice an excess of 'THINGS'. Things that came with exchange of your hard-earned money and precious time. The reality of life is that you don't require 'THINGS' to be happy. Happiness comes from deep inside; its inner work not outer work. In the modern era of toxic consumerism, we are programmed to 'BUY'. We have to 'BUY' to be happy. It's instilled inside our mind through repetitive advertising indirectly or directly that we 'HAVE' to 'BUY' else we will not be part of the smart tribe; whereas it's the entire opposite. We try and fill our emotional voids by shopping, buying, filling our surroundings unnecessarily & then holding on to things with the mindset of usage & memories.

Release this mindset & release these 'THINGS' from your surroundings. The less you own; the better. We are on a transit in this world. Our purpose is not to chain our lives with worldly items only to leave them the second our last breath comes. It's a journey not a stay. Surround yourself with vital things only and focus on raising your vibrations & loving relations. Cherish your relations, yourself & your universe rather than stuffing your physical space with things you don't require.

"Minimalism is not the lack of something. It is the perfect amount of something."

—Nicholas B.

Condition your mind with the right decisions. De-program the 'NEED' of 'BUYING'. Your purchases become 'THINGS' sitting around in your home eventually turning into clutter. Clutter creates confusion, chaos, and restlessness. De-clutter both your physical and mental space in order to function at your optimum pace. Make a commitment with yourself to honor your mother earth, Gaia, this universe, and yourself by following these steps to attract positive energy in your surroundings. Take a walk into your home with a mindset of an outsider who has never been there. Take a good look at everything, every corner. Analyze your

1. Closet
2. Bathroom
3. Kitchen
4. Storage
5. Books & magazines
6. Drawers & cabinets

7.   Your car
8.   Your work-desk
9.   Your home office
10.   Create piles of 'Throw', 'Keep' & 'Sort'.
11.   Re-analyze your pile of 'keep' every week.

Discard everything that's sitting stagnant around you that doesn't serve you and create space for new energy. If you haven't used any of these things in piles since the last 6 months to a year you will never use them. Release these unnecessary things and stagnant energy from your home, office, aura, and experience. When you donate, other souls experience stuff that they could not get otherwise. Your coat could help someone in winters, your chair can help a student study, etc. open up flow – declutter drawers, corners, under the bed, closets. Your donation ritual will attract more and better for you in return in terms of peace & tranquility. You are on a path of transformation & healing. You are entering a better phase of your journey. This is a ritual that is beneficial for your growth.

Detachment is one of the biggest steps of evolvement.

Never get attached to stuff. Change is the only constant in life. Move along with life and change instead of being stagnant. Schedule 3 hours every Saturday morning or Sunday afternoon for de-cluttering. You will be amazed how this ritual and organizing yourself will benefit your life. Simplify your life, your home, your space, and your mind. This ritual will attract new positive energy flow and give you unwavering focus and clarity for your next elevated state & frequency.

Things you can practice daily or weekly to improve the vibrational energy of your physical space.

- Burn sage, incense, oils, or palo santo wood.
- Switch on calming music in your home to elevate the energy.
- Add positive sounds like wind chimes & Tibetan bowls
- Burn nontoxic candles every day around your home (safely)
- In your meditations, Intend and visualize your entire space being filled with the sacred light from your sacred source.
- Open your curtains and allow sunlight to bathe in your interiors and saturate your home with light & love
- Open your windows & doors to allow fresh air to flow through your home.
- Add fresh plants inside your home to purify the air and to bring in life energy.

Feng Shui

Feng Shui is a 5000 years old ancient Chinese ideology that believes the destiny of a person is in direct proportion to his or her environment.

Feng Shui's literal meaning is wind and water. It is a concept to ensure that people live in harmonious surroundings. It is a system of laws that govern the flow of energy in an environment by arrangements of objects in a certain manner. It is a fusion of 'Yin' & 'Yang' energy, the feminine and the masculine synced together in a perfect balance to enhance the flow of 'CHI' (Energy). Feng Shui incorporates the five elements in design and surroundings; water, fire, wood, metal & earth. The ideal balance of these elements creates the perfect surroundings with a powerful & uninterrupted flow of 'Chi'. In the Chinese culture this is the 'Tao'; which translates to "The Way". 'Tao is the way of nature.

Incorporate plants, water fountain, natural stones & crystals, mirrors & lucky objects like 'Lucky Bamboo' plant in your surroundings to activate & ease the flow of 'CHI'.

The 7 Seconds Shock & The 77 Seconds Manifestation

Procrastination is an action where we constantly pay attention to the less important tasks on expense of the vital tasks. Many of us have suffered from this issue at different stages of life. We know what we want, we are aware of what we need to do, yet we procrastinate and delay our important tasks unnecessarily. We avoid the necessary and spend our time doing the unnecessary. This action in itself is a low vibrational state action.

Commit to yourself consciously to take yourself out of this zone and into the optimum, responsible & active zone to combat the procrastination state. The 'Seven Seconds Shock (7SS)' is a ritual that I created to conquer my procrastination zone. Procrastination is a negative state and I wanted to turn this around to a positive productive state. Whenever you feel that you are in a low state of wasting time, delaying important tasks and spending time on mindless activities instead of productive ones, give yourself the 7SS (7 Seconds Shock) out of it.

The 77SS Ritual

Close your eyes & imagine yourself in a high elevated vibrational state. Smile & say to yourself; I AM Powerful & I CAN Turn around This Second. Count 7-6-5-4-3-2-1 and shock yourself out of that mode and immediately get up.

The 77 Seconds Manifestation (77SM)

Focus & faith is powerful. When you intentionally choose a thought and give it your uninterrupted focus and strong faith, your body's energy level will start changing; this is the strongest signal to your infinite intelligence source's guidance system to activate everything in its wisdom, knowledge, and power to manifest your thought into reality.

Focus on your thought for it to activate. 7 seconds of thinking about something will activate a matching vibration to it, and in 77 seconds that thought will start manifesting. Now this vibration that you have conceptualized has become so powerful that it will start manifesting. This is the ripple effect of energy that has initiated in you and will ripple through you in your aura syncing to the universe energy expanding to its power and ultimately attracting a similar energy towards you resulting in the manifestation of your desire. Yes, it's that powerful!

The 77SM Ritual

Breathe deeply. Inhale. Hold. Exhale. Think of a desire and hold it in your mind for 7 long seconds. You have activated a matching vibration to it. Now hold this thought in your mind for the next 77 seconds that's one minute and 17 seconds. Hold it in your mind and feel its reality with emotions and in

203

---

these 77 seconds ritual you have activated its
manifestation.

The Success Secret

To start is ordinary, to finish what you start is extraordinary; which leads to success; hence the Art of Completion.

The difference between ordinary & extraordinary is commitment & persistence. Starting is truly ordinary. All of us start many times, but only a few handful amongst us complete what they start with faith, commitment, and perseverance. The people amongst us who seem lucky, gifted, genius & blessed are in fact the ones who have a clear aim, draft a definitive plan, initiate & see through to its completion without losing faith or getting side-tracked at any cost. Their commitment leads them to success.

There is no other difference between them and ordinary people other than their dire commitment to follow through their plan to its end. Starting something is the easiest task, it's the habit of following through the task to completion is where the success secret lies. Almost all of us have an immense amount of ideas and numerous plans to transform those ideas to reality. Some of us start with tremendous enthusiasm but the very limited amongst us who actually commit themselves to the completion of those tasks are the only ones who are honored with achievement, success & contentment.

Procrastination is the enemy of success. I, myself, have experienced many phases in life where procrastination was the easier task. I suffered because of this habit and now that I learned to overcome this, my intent is to help you not get sucked in by this vicious cycle. Resting and taking a break is completely different than procrastinating and somewhere along the days of our lives we forget the difference and get swallowed by the ease of doing mindless activities instead of diverting & assigning our time to productive tasks, hence the 7SS ritual.

List down your goals and devise plans to achieve your goals as described earlier in this book. After your clear plans, make a commitment to yourself and then honor yourself by achieving the state of completion for your assigned tasks. The key difference between success & failure is something as simple as the 'Art of Completion'.

Bring yourself to the 1% of the population that becomes extraordinary by their commitment, hard work & persistence. To start is ordinary, to finish what you start is extraordinary; hence the success secret.

Part 5

The Secret Aladdin Lamp; Your Subconscious Mind

The subconscious mind is the most powerful instrument in this universe; it is truly the magic lamp that you have in your own hands. The conscious mind is the leader and the subconscious mind is technically the follower. The secret is to find balance between these two. Both are vital in their own manner. The subconscious mind stores all your experiences, words, thoughts & dreams while the conscious mind helps you with your day to day tasks.

"A man is what he thinks about all day long."

–Ralph Waldo Emerson

Nothing is impossible in this world as long as the man has his mind, for the conscious mind controls the subconscious mind and the subconscious mind is the 'POWERHOUSE'. Your subconscious mind is part of the universe in you. It's an unlimited power inside you waiting to be tapped into. It knows no limitations, lack, or restriction. Its greatest attribute is to follow and create. It creates what you want it to create; and your 'want' is directed by your thoughts. "Thoughts" are the magic elixir that direct your subconscious mind to what you desire. Your thoughts and your faith on your thoughts manifest through your mind. Your thoughts can be reformed through meditation. Yes, meditation is the ritual that you can use to program your subconscious mind exactly to what you desire which will result into your conscious mind focusing exactly on specific information, events, and activities that direct you towards your dreams and desires. It's a process that you control and everything is achievable through this magical chain of rituals.

"There is a life force within your soul, seek that life. There is a gem in the mountain of your body, seek that mine. O Traveler, if you are in search of that, don't look outside, look inside yourself and seek that."

—Rumi

Your subconscious mind is truly the magical 'Aladdin lamp' in your own hands to attract and attain anything that you want in this world. It is the gateway to fulfill all your dreams and desires. The understating of this power that lives within your own self will expand your life to unlimited horizons.

"We become what we think about."

—Earl Nightingale

The power of thought is beyond measure provided it comes with faith & conviction. A thought has to be activated with utmost faith in order to become the miracle in your life. A miracle is simply your desire that turns into a thought in your mind with utmost level of faith & conviction. This is the simple yet most powerful formula used by all successful people in this world to achieve and attain anything &everything that they ever desire. Your subconscious mind is your direct connection to your ultimate source.

The power of thought in your subconscious mind is so magnificent that

If you think about failure, your subconscious mind will direct you towards failure

If you think about success, your subconscious mind will direct you towards success

If you think about sadness, your subconscious mind will direct you towards sadness

If you think about happiness, your subconscious mind will direct you towards happiness

---

The 'Infinite Intelligence', your subconscious mind, the 'Divine Power', the 'Eternal Guide', the 'Almighty', the 'Omnipotent', the 'Glorious, whichever words you choose to describe it; flows through every single one of us. It has no limitations or lack. Nothing is Impossible for it. It has the ability is to create; create for us as we want it. It creates according to desire, proportionally to our thoughts, clearly bringing to life every thought that we believe in. Thought plus faith & conviction results in manifestation. Your subconscious mind manifests exactly what you think with conviction.

"The Greatest discovery of my generation is that human beings can alter their lives by altering their attitudes of mind."

—William James

This 'Omnipotent Power' is within each one of us; the power to create exactly what we desire, but we have to learn how to tune in to its frequency and that is done by utmost faith, belief, and conviction. Attunement with the 'Infinite Intelligence' is the magical secret. Rub your 'Aladdin Lamp' by tuning into your subconscious with faith and ask.

Align, Ask, Believe, Allow & Receive.

Allow the 'Law of Attraction' to work in your favor by your thoughts and your faith. Thoughts with Strong faith will create and manifest your desires to reality. Remove all negative thoughts in your system, tune in with your infinite intelligence, believe in the 'Laws of Nature', 'Spiritual Laws', 'Laws of Universe'; then sit back and watch your life change into this magnificent dream giving you everything you have ever desired. The deep understanding of this power and syncing to its frequency with faith will expand your horizons to the unlimited.

Negativity exists in this quantum reality and your mind thinks of negative thoughts throughout the day. The control of those thoughts is the power. All illness, disease, sadness, and negativity are a result of negative thoughts. Intentionally change and redirect your thoughts to positivity, improve the quality of your thoughts, elevate your vibrations, tune into the right frequency, speak the language of the universe which is energy by thinking positively and watch your world transform in front of your eyes.

The universal intelligence, infinite wisdom, your subconscious mind is all within you. You just need to look within, tap into its wisdom, and let it work magical wonders for your life. This is all controlled by the 'Power of Thought'. You create what you think so watch what you think. The power of thought is beyond any power as it syncs and embeds in your subconscious mind and makes it create. Your subconscious mind knows no difference between reality, and imagination. It creates for you as per your dominant thoughts and feelings. Be extremely vigilant in your thoughts and meditate every single day of your life, morning, and evening to give the visualization, affirmations, gratitude, and imagery with emotions to your infinite intelligence so it responds and creates accordingly.

It is true that there is a power, purely magical, enchanting, and infinite, within you. You can tune in with this power and make it work for your advancement exactly the way you desire. Keep in mind that this power cannot differentiate between good and evil. It will create as you desire so make sure your intentions, thoughts, and dreams are positive and with goodwill as they are the only ones that give unlimited abundance. Evil intentions can be achieved but will result in karma hence destruction so watch your thoughts and ask for only good as this is the law of the spiritual world.

The times that our desires are not being manifested is the time to analyze our level of faith and conviction or that particular desire. If we desire something and then get into a negative spiral of thoughts like "This can never happen", "I'm not worth it", "I know my luck is not that good" etc. that particular desire will never manifest as you are questioning the infinite intelligence power. Change your thoughts right away to "I am blessed to receive the best", "I know that infinite intelligence is working for me and making all that I desire come true". "My life is guided and directed by the 'Divine Order' and my life is circulated by the divine love and abundance flows to me as I am a magnet to all kinds of positivity". Practice more positive affirmations rather than negative, denying thoughts. Learn to be aware of any negative thought, delete it at the onset, and change the direction and energy immediately to positive thoughts with white light beaming.

Belief is the foundation to tap into your subconscious mind. Any thought that emerges in your mind powered by faith, belief, and conviction will manifest as this is the law. Believe that you will succeed and you will. Believe that you will fail and you will. Believe that you will be rich and you will. Believe that you will be poor and you will. Believe that you will get sick and you will. Believe that you will attain perfect health and you will. The power is in your belief as it endorses your thought in your subconscious mind for it to start manifesting. The dominant thoughts always manifest. Manifestation occurs with the conception of thought powered by faith and belief. Be aware of your thoughts as your subconscious mind is all-powerful in creation. Use this power to attain all that you have ever desired by 'THINKING' with 'FAITH' about all that you have ever desired.

You have the power to rise above any circumstance, any problem, any issue, any negativity that you are experiencing in life by tapping into this powerful source within you; your subconscious mind. You can change your reality and overcome lack, limitation, poverty, sadness, illness, inferiority, depression, anxiety, fear, etc. with the power of positive thoughts endorsed by very strong faith. We have hundreds of examples around us of people who rose from, illness, poverty, lack, limitations, fear, etc. just by tapping into their infinite source, their subconscious mind.

It is true that every circumstance and event in your life is a result of your own thoughts, that's how powerful it all is. It's the 'Law of Attraction' that operates within us. We attract exactly what we think consciously. You are literally a result of your own beliefs and thoughts. From this day onwards accept the responsibility of elevating the quality of your thoughts and focus on thinking only positive thoughts backed up by faith and conviction. Emotionally feeling the authenticity of all that you desire through thoughts, visualizations, affirmations, and meditations and watch how your life starts to transform right in front of your eyes.

"A man's life is what his thoughts make of it."

—Marcus Aurelius

Look at people around you. Most of them are not aware of the subconscious mind; hence their life is directed completely by circumstances and the result of their unguarded thoughts. They all have absolutely no idea of this infinite power that resides within them. You are chosen to rise above the mediocracy of all this and take control of your life. Take this moment to analyze your desires, dreams, and goals. Are they sacred, are they positive, pure, good and radiate light? You are worthy of all abundance, wealth, prosperity, health, love, peace, joy, happiness, serenity and wisdom that you desire but it all has to follow three simple rules;

1. They have to be with goodwill and good intentions
2. They won't cause any harm to humanity, earth, or the spirit world; or attain any evil intentions.
3. Your dreams and desires must have a way to be of a great source to humanity in any way possible.

Evil intentions can also be answered by your subconscious mind but will result in karma allowing evil to direct itself towards you as well. So be extremely vigilant with your thoughts as with great power comes greater responsibility. If the infinite intelligence is unfolding its secret to you, it expects you to handle it with the utmost sacred, positive, and pure intentions.

Your subconscious mind works 24/7 with the accumulation of thoughts that you have presented it with. The best way to infuse and saturate your subconscious mind with the positive thoughts yielding to your desires and dreams is through meditation which includes affirmations and visualization. Meditation is the art of silencing the conscious mind while embedding the right thoughts in your subconscious mind. Meditation is the tool which gives you control over your thoughts and ultimately helps you in reaching your destiny. Your conscious mind is an instrument that directs your day to day activities and is equally important to your life whereas the subconscious mind dictates and directs your destiny. Both these minds have equally vital responsibilities and the successful person finds balance in operating these minds. The conscious mind keeps us sane and the subconscious mind keeps us directed towards our goals and dreams.

You are a unique soul because no one has the thought pattern that you have and you will create and manifest as per your evolvement, desires & vibrational level. You are different from any soul on this earth and beyond as you have your own unique and special mind and thought process. You are like no other and there is no one like you. If you would understand this little miracle deeply you can achieve anything beyond words.

Search intentionally for quiet moments throughout your day and in those silent moments interact with your powerful subconscious mind by acknowledging its presence and power. It can guide you miraculously and align you with your purpose, your path. You must deeply understand the invincible power of a single thought, how it carves you into who you are, how it directs your life every single day, and how it manifests exactly what you strongly believe in. How it alters circumstances and brings in your experience everything that you secretly wish for with conviction, good or bad. How it aligns the events of the universe to make sure you receive what you ask for. It has incomprehensible power and you are aware of it now and exactly how it works.

"Self-control is strength, right thought is mastery; calmness is power."

—James Allen

We must protect ourselves from any negative thoughts that may enter our minds. We should refuse to entertain such thoughts and transient them with strong positive thoughts immediately. As the mind creates everything that is sent towards it with faith, you have to intentionally control this pattern and overlap it immediately. You want only positive thoughts that work towards your dreams. There is no such thing as fate and luck; we create as we want. Every single thing that you have around you is the creation of thoughts that you have had in the past. If you want better, upgrade your thoughts.

If you want your life to be filled with love, achievement, prosperity, happiness, joy, peace, success, and health, you will learn to abandon every single negative thought as soon as you become aware of that thought entering your mind.

If you understood the power of a single thought and its ripple effect, you would never let a negative thought stay in your mind for a second.

Plato, Michelangelo, Leonardo Da Vinci, Einstein, Shakespeare, Tesla, Edison, all knew the magical power of the subconscious mind and attained the alignment to retrieve the utmost knowledge, art, and skills they desired. You are no different from them since you now know the secret. Great genius lies in each one of us just waiting to be discovered and used. All we have to do is acknowledge and tap into the great power, align and sync with its magnificence, believe that it is enchanting yet true, resulting in opening the doors of infinite wisdom to our lives achieving everything that we have ever dreamt of.

Tune in to the frequency of the universe, converse with the universe in the language that it understands; which is energy, vibrations, and frequency. Tune in and open the world of infinite possibilities manifesting everything that you have ever desired.

Health, wealth, abundance, prosperity, happiness, wellness, peace, all these words have tremendous power and strength. Anchor your thoughts around them and around words like them that flow with your desires & goals; resultantly circumstances and events corresponding and aligning to these words will be initiated and manifested in your life from your never-ending source power.

Words are Spells (Literally)

We speak approximately 600-7000 words in a day. Each spoken word transforms into sound, vibration & frequency in the universal language hence attaining the power as to how energy manifests itself into reality.

"In the beginning was the Word." (John 1:1-3)

Words are more powerful than swords as they can heal you or harm you at the deepest core of your being. Every word is a sound frequency possessing hidden knowledge good or evil as per intention. They carry the frequency which is the language of the universe. Information is carried through these word frequencies and transported to us via sounds when we hear them. Sound is a natural source used by nature and sacred geometry, creating wonders. Sound controls and directs energy and frequency to create sacred geometry. Watch this video on YouTube to decipher the power of sound energy to create sacred geometry. "Cymatics: Sacred Geometry Formed by sound".

Words spoken and words heard, both become sounds transforming into frequency, absorbed by your aura, soul; and ultimately your subconscious mind. Words are the tools of communication to release energy and direct it to attain desired results consciously and unconsciously. The sooner you realize the power of words, sounds, frequencies, energy, and vibrations; the sooner you will rise above this artificial controlled matrix freeing your mind, body, and soul achieving spiritual freedom.

Speaking negatively about your experience, your day, your things, your environment, or you, as a habit, to gain sympathy or for fun is extremely harmful. Your body doesn't know the difference and your mind will grasp and store every word as a suggestion and start working on it. Words are literally energy spells. Change the way you speak about yourself and change your life in exact proportion to your words, thoughts, emotions & faith.

Never use words, statement or phrases like 'I can't', 'I won't', 'I don't', 'I will never', 'I'm not worth it', 'this will never come to me', 'I'm unlucky', 'I hate this', etc. These are low-frequency negative thoughts and low vibrational words; they have no purpose in your life and your journey any more.

"Each word that you speak carries consciousness – more than that, carries intelligence – and therefore, is an intention that shapes light."

—*Gary Zukav*

Words, when spoken, are sending energy and vibrations to the earth's magnetic field and this energy field creates your reality. You cast a spell (literally) each time you say any word (s) positive or negative. Words are hypnotic to our mind unconsciously. Your awareness about this is the most powerful spiritual defense that you have.

The language of the universe is based on frequency, sound, vibration, and sacred geometry. This language is the most powerful system ever.

If you would understand how powerful your thoughts and words are, you wouldn't think of a single negative thought or speak one negative word in your entire life. Your thoughts and your words become your reality. Read that again because it's far more real than you can ever perceive.

Your thoughts and your words become your reality.

When you are talking to yourself and you say, 'I am so stupid what was I thinking". Your subconscious mind picks the word 'stupid' and stores it. You say, "I always have bad luck, I will always be a failure". Your subconscious mind will store the words 'bad luck' & 'failure'. From this moment onwards throughout the day, months, and years to come, your subconscious brain will only direct your attention to everything that resonates with words like 'stupid', 'bad luck' and 'failure'. Ultimately making you see, choose, and live a low vibrational life. This is how powerful your thoughts and words are. Until you reprogram your subconscious mind to think differently it will keep doing this. Now imagine how many negative thoughts and words you have experienced since the past years. The good news is that you can reprogram your mind to a new state and to a better upgraded future.

Be vigilant and mindful of your thoughts and the words that you speak. Pay attention to the way you talk about yourself and the way you talk about other people. This is the first and foremost way to keep your vibration high, by keeping your words and your thoughts positive, happy, constructive, productive, and kind. Chose only powerful, positive & productive thoughts and words so you sustain your high vibrational status, and ultimately your reality shapes into exactly what your goals and dreams are. The entire universe is energy and when you learn how to control and direct this energy, unlimited power comes in your own hands. If you want to protect your physical body then intentionally guard your 'THOUGHTS'. Negative thoughts such as jealousy, hatred, evil, malice, disappointments, sadness, envy, destroy your body and take away health, happiness, and vitality. They strip your body of positivity and light and fill your body with darkness hence on setting disease and degeneration of your body.

Let's simply work in accordance to the highest law, 'The Law of Nature', 'Law of Universe', 'Law of Spirit' & 'Law of Infinite', which magnitudes to such an extent that the law of the physical real world seems almost insignificant in comparison to it. Let's tune in to the frequency of the ultimate vibration and align our life according to its worth. Your conscious mind is the foundation of your daily life. It controls the order, routine, and sanity of your soul. It works with your subconscious mind keeping you sane and normal. Balance in controlling both these aspects of your mind. Your conscious mind and subconscious mind work in a circle of union. Any imbalance would create insanity or obsession wither way. Herein lies the secret of the genius.

Flood your subconscious mind with all your intentions, positive thoughts, and desired dreams with emotions. Have utmost faith that whatever you desire is manifesting and your conscious mind will work like a miracle focusing and guiding you towards your dreams.

You must trust and have faith that a power much greater than you is directing all your efforts in result of your wishes and prayers. You don't need to worry about the ways and means of how it will all come together and materialize into your reality. The Universe and its magical powers will synchronize and orchestrate every sequence of events in accordance to the direction of your thoughts and wishes. You must believe and have strong conviction of the manifestation of your desires by your subconscious mind; your 'Eternal Power' source. As it will take its own time, directions, ways, and means to bring forth to you exactly what you desire. Throughout this journey, you may be faced with negative events but you must trust the 'Infinite Intelligence' and its power of direction and redirection according to your desires. It will take paths and ways best suited to accomplish the task that you have assigned to it. Trust with conviction that it will achieve it the right and best way for you.

What you may think of as a negative event may be a blessing in disguise as the infinite intelligence is redirecting and realigning everything in your experience to manifest your dreams, desires, and goals.

By the power of intentionally choosing our THOUGHTS every single day, we are training ourselves to accept only love, compassion, kindness, joy, happiness, abundance, health, vitality, prosperity, vigor, and constant evolvement towards improving ourselves. We are teaching our minds to direct all its energy towards achieving our dreams and desires manifesting all that we have ever wanted in our lives. Simultaneously we are training our minds to reject everything negative, evil, and wrong.

Learn to trust your subconscious mind completely and have faith that every delay and every obstacle is an opportunity, a redirection, and a blessing in disguise. No moment is wasted; every single thing that comes into your experience is preparing you for the next moment and its significance will unfold eventually, learn to 'TRUST'. Turn all your negatives to positives in your own mind. All negatives are only detours and redirections, nothing more. Evil is an illusion, don't accept anything evil, sad, negative, or wrong in your experience. Even if it comes refuse to accept its presence and think of it as just an illusion. Whatever you give focus and energy to will expand; choose wisely.

When you trust your subconscious mind and embed in it intentionally all thoughts and emotions that you desire then your worries end as the infinite intelligence and its powers take over. You align and sync with the immortelle power and let it direct you towards your goals, dreams, and desires. The universal mind knows best and takes perfect steps towards your goals with infinite wisdom and the powers of the universe. Imagine the power of thought that 80% of all diseases occur in the mind and then inhibit your body. Disease is a product of negative mental thoughts and low vibrational energy. All great healers knew the secret that the body and mind are one.

A Secret

When you align yourself with the universe you will see a drastic improvement in your desires and dreams. If your desires and dreams are more towards the worldly things then you may need to move yourself to a higher vibration as there is no infinite pleasure in worldly desires. A nice car or a beautiful home may bring you joy for some time but it won't fulfill the void inside you. Strive and desire towards betterment and benefit of humanity and all your worldly desires will manifest themselves as by the 'Law of mutual gain' when you desire the prosperity and benefits of others, the same is sent towards you. At that moment you will enjoy all worldly desires with a deep fulfilled heart and a feeling of contentment as your direction is not just worldly it constitutes the benefit of humanity; hence the universe will respond in abundance.

How can you benefit Humanity and make it prosper?

There is no such thing as 'Independence', it is a man-made illusion for secrecy and isolation. It is indeed the idea of the evil as it knows the power you have and attain when you align with your source. Everything in the universe is interlinked and intertwined. When we isolate ourselves and sync out from its vibrations we are alone and we suffer tremendously. A soul all by himself, alone is a minor speck in the universe exposed to all negativity and evil, whereas the same soul synced, aligned and attuned with the universal power has the power of the entire universe within itself.

He who syncs with the 'Ultimate Source' is blessed as the 'Eternal Source Energy' aligns with it and moves with power resulting in all actions being rewarded and blessed. These genius, evolved souls achieve more in minutes than the average person achieves in a lifetime because of their knowledge, faith, and conviction. Their entire movement and activity are guided by the wisdom and infinite intelligence of the universe.

They are directed and guided towards their paths with protection and intelligence by the universal mind itself; hence they are known as a genius. All they have mastered is the art of using their subconscious mind's power, aligning themselves to their source, having sacred positive intentions towards the service of humanity and the entire universe power is at their disposal. This power guides them and they achieve everything plus dignity in this physical world.

The law of mutual exchange works like a miracle for the same reason. When you find your purpose, skills, and traits and uncover your potential, you must use it in a way that benefits humanity and ultimately the universe. The law of nature in return blesses you with all that you have ever wanted and beyond. Anything that is service to the universe is excellent and will reward you a million-fold. It's such a simple secret and you have it now to utilize it to achieve all that you have ever desired while making this world a better place. This fulfillment of desires and dreams comes with contentment and peace.

If you base your life dreams, desires, passion, and security on material world possessions like money, you will soon experience and realize how invaluable money is. The actual treasure lies in the attainment, attunement, and alignment with the universal power. That is the security that you should strive for as it is abundant and endless.

Directing your faith from the universe to money is exactly where the disconnection arises. Prosperity, abundance, wealth, infinite gains, service of humanity, benefit to fellows, and everything in the law of mutual gain cycle, are all sacred laws of the universe, the spiritual world, and the source energy, God. Whereas the pursuit of worldly possessions and money is an act of being selfish, senseless, temporary, and is truly degrading to the soul and spirit of man. This approach will always be short-lived and will always come without peace and contentment.

Upgrade your thought process from money to service. How can you serve humanity? Your inner trait is to create not compete. Create things that offer knowledge, prosperity, and betterment to humanity. Produce and sell goods and products that are pure and beneficial to humanity. Create opportunities and jobs for people. Identify better ways and manners to offer goods and services to people for their benefit and make their lives easier. Be of service in any way or by any platform.

If you are not clear of your purpose and gift that will serve humanity then with sacred intentions throw this question to your subconscious mind at night and let it answer you in the coming days and moments. You may be skilled in inspiring, guiding, building, painting, writing, developing, attaining, creating, producing, organizing, or something else that you may not be personally aware of. Your source wisdom will guide you and direct you towards it when you 'ASK'. When that special skill is unveiled to you, take that opportunity and be of service through your skill, and as per the law of mutual gain the universe will shower itself through all blessings that you have ever desired. This mutual equation of service and gain will bring peace, fulfillment, contentment, abundance, prosperity, and wealth in your life experience.

Don't worry about how it will all work out. When you desire it, the universe will bring to your experience all knowledge, tools, techniques, methods, workforce, organization, and formation in your experience, guiding you seamlessly towards its manifestation.

"Ask. Believe. Receive."

—Rhonda Byrne (The Secret)

You may choose platforms like writing, farming, education, technology, industry, manufacturing, export, import, arts, sciences, or any other, In the end, the result of all should be benefit, service, welfare, and prosperity of humanity, society, and universe.

"There is a tide in the affairs of men

which taken at the flood leads on to Fortune

omitted, all the voyage of their life

is bound in shallows and in miseries."

—William Shakespeare

The Glide Vantage

Life on earth is a very short period of your soul's stay. It's not to be taken as seriously and intensely as we do. It's to be felt, experienced, and learned from to flow through. We are not to get attached to anything in this world yet we attach ourselves physically, emotionally & mentally to almost everything. We grasp and cling to people & things desperately not realizing that everything is in flow within itself and around us. Everything is in momentum and there is no reason to attach ourselves to anything. Relations, material things, money, everything is in flow, it will come and it will leave when its time is up. The secret is to detach ourselves completely from anything that is from this world and flow through this journey on earth like water in a stream cleansing ourselves with every experience and moment and moving forward without strings. When we attach ourselves, our flow is affected, our energy is halted, our frequency is disturbed and our vibrations start lowering, making our life stagnant.

Learn to 'Glide' through life, its moments, its experiences, relations, and all worldly matters. Gliding is to move smoothly in a continuous flow & motion, without getting attached and accepting the fact that everything around us is temporary. Life is a blend of happiness &

sadness, positivity & negativity, right & wrong, birth & death; these are facts and we all experience everything on our own timings in our own way, yet the goal is to not cling to any of this whether good or bad, acknowledge, experience, feel but move on. Gliding through life without anything affecting you in any manner is the art of spirituality. You experience good & bad but you know it's temporary so you keep gliding to experience the next moment.

When we hold on to things, experiences, worldly matters, or people, we get stuck and our life halts stagnating our energy. Our soul becomes caged. Every experience or emotion we cling to ties a knot within our energy system and blocks the flow. Our souls are not to be caged but to glide freely through this journey on earth to ascend to the next dimension eventually. We are here to learn our lessons not to stagnate ourselves with worldly matters.

Flow is the master key to spirituality, to ascend, to raise your vibrations. Glide through it all rather than clinging to unnecessary temporary thoughts, emotions & experiences.

The idea is to live through this world with the physical body but not mental attachment. You are an eternal being passing through this temporary journey. Be so liberated that nothing controls you. Encompass your entire being in pure compassion, gentleness & love. Let go of any selfish or worldly interest from your being. Detach your soul from any stress, worry, anxiety & pain. You are passing through this world. In an experience of happiness, cherish yet glide, in an event of sadness, feel the emotion yet glide through it. Don't stop, don't halt, don't engage, and don't stay there. Keep moving through the experience with a relaxed aura. This world is not meant to be attached to, it's meant to be experienced with the flow. Let things come & go, let events orchestrate in front of your eyes, watch, feel, experience, learn, and let go. This is the art to live & to ascend in spirituality. Let nothing encompass your being in any extreme. Experience happiness & flow through it, experience sadness & flow through it. Keep all your energy centers flowing and 'Glide' your way through every experience so you are fully present for the next experience.

Radiate peace, glory & love, keep your words short & meaningful, be inspiring & mystical, let your company purify other souls, illuminate light from your being, be so contented within yourself that you become a source of inspiration for others.

This 'Gaia', this earth, this universe, your subconscious; none of these are in any hurry or stress, yet everything happens in a flow. Let go, trust, and glide through life. Every emotion that you have stored in your being becomes a knot and stores itself, only to come out periodically to inflict pain and then go back inside your being.

Slowly these knots increase and your energy system becomes clogged and blocked. These unfinished emotions and energy patterns start affecting the course of your life as you descend towards lower vibrational state; you start attracting lower vibration experiences ultimately falling into a deep state of depression, anxiety, and loss of interest in living life.

Untie these knots by opening your heart and letting go. Remove these negative energy blocks by acknowledging the experiences and letting them leave your aura through meditations & rituals of forgiveness and healing. Intentionally feel your energy centers beaming with light, imagine the flow of energy through you. Detach yourself from any worldly matters, relations, or emotions.

For any future experiences, learn to acknowledge, experience, feel & glide through it. Don't stay there, flow through life.

Any memory, emotion, experience, past that comes up, immediately relax your aura, unclench your teeth, take a deep breath, relax your shoulders and slowly open your heart, imagine love and light radiating through it and slowly let go. Don't hold on to it, let it pass through your being and leave your aura, forever. Throughout your life, the pain will resurface. Don't push it back inside. Let it surface, heal it, and release it. When you practice this, you will be in control of your energy power, your emotions, and your strength. This is called being centered, being in control. This is you with your powerful subconscious mind, your omnipotent power with you against the worldly matters.

Let's stop fighting with life, let's stop resisting, controlling & predicting life. Choose to live in flow, live in love, and let everything glide. Once you are centered and in control, similar events, people, and experiences that would have completely demolished your being in the past can come and go from your life leaving you in perfect harmony, peace, and in control. You are here to experience it all not to get attached with any of it. It's all temporary, almost an illusion. There is a lesson behind every experience, focus on the lesson not the experience. Life will surround you with experiences necessary for your growth nudging you towards your purpose here. Every experience is for your growth, purification, ascension, and re-direction.

Glide through life instead of fearing it, fighting it, resisting it, or controlling it. Disengage your soul from any worldly matter, don't participate in any unnecessary energy draining event; just flow right through it.

Life is a series of experiences; a journey of love and pain, a path of learning & creation between your first breath and your last breath; that's all life is. You are here to experience everything for your spiritual growth. Let go of resistance and clinging. You arrived in this dimension alone and you will leave alone from here. No one and nothing is going with you when you leave. None of us know when our last breath is going to be, yet we are constantly engulfed with stress, fear, hatred, and competition. Live each day as it's your last. Live each moment as it's your last moment, take each breath as it's your last. Cherish this life and ascend yourself to higher vibrations to glide through this life effortlessly and with a smile.

Your choices every day define the course of your life. Attachment to anything in this life is a waste of your time and energy as everything is flowing; choose to glide. You have to pass this time on this earth. Rise above the worldly experiences and ascend yourself to a state of bliss so nothing that happens whether elation or adversity can alter your state of being. You experience and flow right through it.

7 Laws of the Universe

Understanding the powerful laws of the universe will transform the way you look at the universe & your life. Your current life is a manifestation of these laws working exactly how you have been thinking and attracting. You are the co-creator of your life. The powers you have are beyond measure. Understanding the laws and their powerful reality can make you turn your life around. Once you are aware of the laws and their functions, you can co-create your life from this point onwards exactly how you desire.

1. The Law of Vibration

We are all one; the universe is a unified entity that includes us. Everything around us is a part of our being. We are all energy and connected in vibrations. "I am" is us and the universe. Our entire being is connected to the universal energy. Hence every action we take has an effect on the universal oneness. We are all one and a part of the 'Divine Oneness'.

Everything around us is energy; we are the same. The world we see & the unseen universe; it is all ruled by vibration, ranging from the lowest frequency to the highest frequency. The reality that we are currently experiencing individually is the result of these vibrations, initiated by thought. When we commit &

consciously make an effort to raise our vibration, our reality immediately starts changes attracting those things & people that are beneficial for us on our path. Commit your life to incorporate the seven zones explained to increase your vibrations & frequency. An instant way to elevate your vibration is through 'Giving' & 'Gratitude'.

2. The Law of Correspondence

Everything in this universe has a positive and a negative. There is always the day and night. They are dire opposites of each other yet perform their specified tasks in order to support each other. There is always a 'Yin' and 'Yang'; a low & a high. In our daily life when events & situations around us seem like they are flowing in a negative manner, we must recall the law of correspondence; which explains that a negative situation is not the opposite of positive; In fact, it is a part of the synchronized positive coming your way. You may not see it right away but the situation is negative to clear out paths for the positive that you have been thinking & attracting. When you find yourself in a situation that you don't want to be in; instead of going in a negative emotional spiral; use it to practice the art of raising your vibration. This will change your reality and attract what you desire. Everything around us is in constant motion and on a continuum, there is no positive without a negative, no happiness without sadness, no elevation without an experience of a downward spiral. It's our attitude towards the experience that matters. The law of correspondence explains that the contrast is needed for you to realize the value of the opposite. Sometimes you have to experience darkness before you realize exactly how much light is needed to get the clarity you need at that particular moment.

3. The Law of Cause and Effect

Every single thought we have and every single action that we consciously or unconsciously perform has a reaction. We reap what we sow; our reality right now is exactly what our thoughts & actions were in the past years. We experience exactly what we have asked for. It's a constant circle of events. Some may call it karma; some call it blessings. The law of cause & effect is a simple rule that the universe runs by. Whatever you think & do is exactly what you receive back.

There is an equal & opposite reaction to every single action. The intention behind every action determines the reaction's karma. Past actions determine your current reality. The potential energy & vibration hidden behind every action in our lives becomes kinetic. Every action initiates a chain of events that is a reaction; hence the law of cause & effect.

4. The Law of Compensation

Whatever we think, we attract. When we think we create an action manifesting the exact thought. Action is our thoughts in motion. It's all energy, frequency & vibrations collectively performing for us. We should consciously direct our emotions & focus our thoughts and actions on the things we want in our lives. The miraculous trait of this Law is that it initiates exactly as the thought initiates. Once we exude a certain thought, energy, or vibration, the universe has no choice but to respond with a corresponding frequency. This is why it is extremely important to be conscious of your thoughts all day. One negative thought or emotion will activate the universe to compensate you with the similar frequency experience and event. The reality which we manifest is a direct compensation for our vibration, frequency, energy, thoughts, emotions, and actions. It's a default setting by which the universe works so choose your thoughts & perform your actions wisely; attract better. If you find yourself in a negative spiral; immediately snap out of it with the **77SS (7 second shock ritual)** and enter the positive zone to counter the situation and attract what you need to attract.

5. The Law of Attraction

The strongest law is the law of attraction; you attract what you think. You attract what you believe and you attract what you say. Your thoughts & words are vibrational frequency. Every vibration is matched with its proportionate frequency. If you are constantly in a negative mode your life will become a spiral of negativity as that's what you are attracting. If you are positive all the time, you will attract similar frequency & events following it. The universal 'Law of Attraction' is technically in your own hands. You can make it work magnetically for yourself by actively thinking & speaking only that you desire & how you want your life to be. You manifest exactly what you want. You attract exactly what you desire consciously or subconsciously. You make your reality by your thoughts & words. You may call it divine timing or coincidence, but every thought, word, and feeling are a seed and will germinate into your reality.

6. The Law of Rhythm

Everything around you in this universe moves in a rhythmic poetry. The vibrations around us are always in a pendulum moving from side to side. As in the pendulum's reality, everything that swings to the left must swing to the right for the continual rhythm & flow. The energy is never chaotic; it's always in an order, hence the 'Law of Rhythm'. The entire existence in this world is involved in a synchronized movement, flowing back & forth. There is a hidden pattern & rhythm; even in chaos. You notice the pattern & order in the day & night, the seasons, the cycles of life, birth & death. Everything is in constant movement and in a certain rhythm. Hence any particular time of your life will never stay like that forever. What seems to be random is in reality following a pattern. Everything changes; that's the universal law. The key is to master the balance between each side of the pendulum. What seems like chaos to you is an orchestrated and orderly chain of events by the universe. It's the rearrangement & redirection.

"Everything flows, out & in; everything has its tides; all things rise & fall; the pendulum-swing manifests in everything; the measure of the swing to the right is the measure of the swing to the left; rhythm compensates."

—Kybalion

7. The Law of Belief

We do not believe what we see; we rather see what we internally & strongly believe to be true. The universe doesn't give you what you want or desire. It gives you exactly what you believe in.

Our beliefs are simply perspectives that have been programmed & conditioned within our minds over the course of our life through experiences, events, past, memories, circumstances & thinking/ overthinking. We attract what we believe in. Our internal faith & belief system governs every aspect of our life. Our life is a clear manifestation of our beliefs. Whatever we consciously or unconsciously believe to be true is exactly what manifests into our reality. Beliefs are only illusions and can be altered consciously with effort & commitment.

Evolve, alter & improve your beliefs & strongly work on authenticating them within your heart & soul; then notice your reality changing in your favor. Reject the limiting beliefs inside you to weaken their control over your reality & life. Add strong emotions to your upgraded belief system to attract your dreams. This is transformation.

"As a man thinketh, so he becomes."

—James Allen

Your Genesis; Rebirth

You have a goldmine within you, an endless treasure inside you to tap into for everything that you have ever desired. Courage, love, strength, dedication, health, healing, harmony, positivity, happiness, success, abundance, joy, contentment; everything is inside you. Knowledge, awareness & balance of your conscious and subconscious mind is your magical power; your rebirth, your genesis. A giant magnet will attract and lift ten times its own weight but if you demagnetize it, it will not even be able to attract or lift a needle. Your vibrations are the exact phenomenon.

Your infinitely powerful subconscious mind has enchanted powers, clairvoyance, psychic traits, spiritualistic vision, and clairaudience. It has the power to bring you wisdom and knowledge of the entire universe in one second at your will as it is void of worldly limits. It is limitless and is free from the concept of space, time, and dimension. It is not controlled by the matrix. Use it wisely to serve humanity and to make a difference. Abundance, prosperity, happiness, contentment & success will be attracted towards you as a by-product of your sincere efforts.

Your life is a miracle and it is in the flow of the divine order. Heal, transform, rise, advance, grow, and ascend to the limitless universal energy. Fall in

love with yourself. You are the creator of your own happiness. You are a co-creator in this universe.

Spend time with your 'Sacred Source', talk to it, ask, instruct, analyze with it. Let it guide you to the best for you. Every morning and every night before sleeping, initiate a conversation inside your mind with your infinite intelligence. Activate your power source with tasks so it can start bringing the answers to you and direct you accordingly. Throughout your day, on multiple occasions, ask for moments of guidance. Take quiet moments here and there throughout your day to tap into this eternal wisdom source for the right directions. Then rest in the feeling of strong faith and deepest conviction that all your life is taken care of by your source's wisdom.

You are not dependent on any other soul on this earth for happiness, health, abundance, contentment, security, prosperity, strength, or peace. It is all within you. Strive to attain all of this yourself and you will. You can overcome any weakness, sadness, negativity, helplessness, sickness, fear, pain, and low vibrations; all by yourself. You are the one you've been waiting for all your life. Look inwards for the solution to everything. Trust yourself; you are enough; as you are the universe.

"The secret to flight: Don't flap your wings so hard, it only exhausts you. Close your eyes, lean into the currents, and say yes. Let the wind raise you higher and higher. So easy; that's what

eagles do and yes this is the secret to life as well."

—Anonymous

Suffering doesn't go, its form changes. It's when and how you learn to deal with it is the lesson and power. Come to peace with pain. Change is the only constant and change is never comfortable. It challenges the familiarity to the unknown suddenly. Experience it, feel it & then choose to glide through it without staying there. Life will become a free-flowing liberating experience. You are not here on this earth to suffer, you are here to flow, learn, create, ascend, assist, and connect to your source.

Meditation strengthens your core, your deep inner self. Meditation centers your being and calms your mind. It unlocks your subconscious self and syncs you back to it ultimately taking you back to your eternal source energy. If you want to stay there in that ecstasy learn to be happy and to glide through life. Once you commit yourself to be done with the temporary worldly affairs, you will find the eternal divine energy and infinite love within yourself. This path is of pure love, liberation, freedom, nirvana, ecstasy, contentment, bliss, and serenity.

Keep your soul at peace by choosing not to react but respond to life, its events & people around you. A reaction comes from ego and response comes from the mind, but something farther than that is compassion in response. Choose the latter as it will continue the peace in your heart. When you make the choice of responding to a positive or negative event, keep in mind that by this initiative you are choosing to engage in the other side's energy. This connection may alter your frequency as per the other side's vibration. Choose how, when, and who to respond very wisely, keeping the fact in mind that initiating this may lower your vibration as you have to be at the same wavelength to establish communication.

Your spiritual ascension is learning to glide through this temporary life finding your inner eternal source energy, God, universe, love & to flow through this life without getting attached to stress, fear, problems, or even too much happiness. Everything is in constant movement and will pass.

"For a star to be born, there is one thing that must happen; a nebula must collapse. So collapse. Crumble. This is not your destruction. This is your birth."

— n.t.

I believe we go through 7 major events during our average lifetime on this earth. The first is our birth, followed by other experiences and rebirths that change our lives forever. We come out different from every incident; a genesis every time into a new & evolved being; if we choose the path of positivity. This is a ritual of continual genesis to transform us; only to align us back to where we belong.

AGING; and the fear behind it.

We start aging the moment we arrive in this world. Every moment after that is aging our body. Our mind and soul are ageless. Our mind is a result of our constant drive to learn & be creative. Life is a spiritual journey and is eternal. We are spiritual beings having a human experience and once this experience ends we transfer to another realm, dimension, or state. This is a journey and age is a number. We are as old as our mind perceives. Our subconscious mind never gets old, our body starts aging as soon we take our first breath on this earth.

Aging is not the years gone but the wisdom attained, the knowledge acquired, the evolvement, the alignment with your source energy, and the advancement in the spiritual realm.

Aging is the awareness that we gain with every experience and moment. Our attitude determines our age, our mindset determines our age, our goals determine our age, our drive and willpower determine our age, our purpose determines our age, our choices determine our age and our physical health determines our age.

Age is in our own hands. There can be a healthy, super active, goal-oriented, evolved, happy 70-year-old feeling and looking like a 50-year-old and there can be a pessimistic, unhealthy, non-active individual who has no goals and purpose who may look like a 70-year-old due to his lifestyle choices. Age is in your own hands and mind. Some people are old and miserable at 30 and some people are positive, active, full of life, vibrant and vivacious at age 70. It all depends on your lifestyle, your thought process, your choices & your priorities.

You start to deteriorate when you lose interest in life, when you have no goals or purpose to wake up to, when you are out of alignment with your source, when you stop dreaming, when you "give-up", when you lose hope, when you surround yourself with pessimism and negativity and when you "retire" mentally to live. This is when your mind gets the signal to start the degeneration process; hence your immune system starts deteriorating inviting diseases.

Think of the empty nest years or the retirement years as an opportunity to rediscover life your way. Do the things you've always wanted to do but never found the time to. Take your mind back to your early years and find yourself, uncover everything that you always desired to learn and do but never found the courage or time to do. Take up the dancing lessons, learn golf, start swimming, learn how to paint, start your herb garden, create a recipe cook book, initiate a social networking group of your friends and coordinate travels and events etc.

Enjoy your life to the last breath. Set an example of how a vivacious life is lived for your generation and community. Inspire, rejuvenate, recharge, and transform your mind to live the best years of your life from this moment onwards whether you are 20, 30, 50, and 80. It doesn't matter. Focus on aging spiritually not physically. When you age at the spiritual level you radiate wisdom, light & love.

You are not a number; you are the accumulation of your experiences, your wisdom, your thoughts, your aura, your energy, your frequency, and your vibrations. Celebrate yourself and every breath that you take in his human form. Live and inspire others to live.

Your Avatar

Being spiritual is who we are deep inside. It's time to reclaim our identity. We are sacred source energy. Let's raise our vibrations, connect to our sacred source, and heal this world and universe elevating everyone with us. Our desire, faith & commitment is the initiation process for the universe to manifest all for us. We are vibrational entities in this universe which speak the language of frequency, energy & vibration. Once we 'Align', 'Ask' & 'Allow' our entire physical experience in this world starts changing for the better.

The optimal experience will be for us to surrender and sync to the energy and vibrations of this universe, allowing everything to come into our experience, feeling optimistic and excited, without doubt or fear altering the reception, is the seamless magic formula for creation and manifestation of all our desires by the Universe.

Every thought that occurs in our mind creates a vibration which gets a similar response and attracts a matching vibrational signal from the universe. When we desire something, we raise our vibrations and connect with the universe for the matching vibrational frequency to attract everything we require to manifest our desires. The key to attracting into our experience that which we desire is to attain vibrational syncing

& harmony with exactly what we desire; and the optimum manner to do that is to imagine that we already have it. Our emotions attract the equivalent vibration of the universe; manifesting our desire.

You are the sculptor of your own life, having the power to carve your life exactly how you want it to be. You are a vibrational being having the power to take your energy and elevate it to the level that you want to attract. You are the creator and author of your own life. Your powerful source energy resides inside you waiting to be discovered and directed.

Whatever you give intentional or unintentional attention to, will be returned with a similar experience. Your dominant thoughts endorsed by your faith will manifest. Nothing can come into your experience unless it's been attracted by you yourself. For this reason, you have to guard your thoughts constantly. You are manifesting when you are happy, sad, angry, jealous, peaceful, in gratitude, in appreciation, in awe, in worry, in stress, etc. You are constantly attracting the vibration of what you are experiencing every single moment of your life. Getting stressed, worried, anxious, or sad is using your mind to attract and manifest exactly what you don't want.

Every experience & emotion in your life is a result of your alignment with the respective energy vibration. Watch your thoughts and continuously work on raising your vibrations so you attract the best for yourself. Trust the universe and learn the art of receiving and allowing everything into your life experience seamlessly. Don't resist, trust, have faith, and let it all flow naturally to its poetic rhythm.

You are a spirit having a human experience not a human learning about the spiritual realm. You are a soul here in this dimension to experience this physical world to learn, evolve, attain, and leave when your time is up. Make the best of this experience and leave this dimension with a more powerful, more evolved, more elevated soul.

Your environment becomes you. Be vigilant about what you are watching, listening to, reading, experiencing, eating, your social life, your friends and family that you are surrounded with. All this will become 'YOU'. Everyone around you is having the same experience as you but everyone is at a different vibrational level evolving according to their awareness. We are all co-creators of each other's experiences. We all have our own beliefs, notions, and emotions depending on our evolvement. Compassion, patience, and kindness will help us on this journey to deal with diversity of thoughts and emotions that others are experiencing.

This world is a quantum reality. This diversity and contrast around you helps you in your own direction and gives you clarity of everything that syncs with you and everything that doesn't sync with who you are. Your emotions are the guiding system here. This diversity gives you clarity. When you experience what repulses you or doesn't sync in with you, thank it for its experiences and distance yourself accordingly so your energy can move and elevate with ease.

"What you seek is seeking you."

—Rumi

Whatever you are seeking is already seeking you. All you need to do is match your frequency to your desire's frequency and it will align into your life; effortlessly. Once the seed of desire is placed in your heart it is simultaneously synchronized in this universal frequency to manifest itself for you; should you desire with faith & make an effort. The alignment & manifestation of your dreams depend solely on your effort & desire to sync to the required frequency by elevating your vibrations; committing yourself to follow the disciplined routine explained in the zones.

Another interesting concept is the RRP. Activate the RRP (Reverse receiving process). Whatever you wish to seek; imagine it seeking you. For e.g. you would like your book to heal every soul on this earth, imagine every soul in pain looking for healing & transformation; needing your book. By the law of attraction; those souls in need of healing, guidance & transformation will start advancing towards your book. The universe will choreograph and synchronize it all so beautifully. This is reverse receiving and it completes the circle of allowing. Align, Attract & Allow.

"A wise woman who was traveling in the mountains found a precious stone in a stream. The next day she met another traveler who was hungry, the wise woman opened her bag to share her food. The hungry traveler saw the precious stone and asked the woman to give it to him. She did so without hesitation. The traveler left, rejoicing in his good fortune. He knew the stone was worth enough to give him security for a lifetime. But a few days later he came back to return the stone to the wise woman. 'I've been thinking', he said 'I know how valuable the stone is, but I give it back in the hope that you will give me something even more precious. Give me what you have within you that enabled you to give me this stone.'"

—Zen Tale

Success is not a competition. You are in competition with no one. This universe has unlimited resources enough for all. It creates more in proportion to its soul's desires. Reject the idea of competition or scarcity and embrace the thought of creation. Create the best that you can, cherish who you are, and celebrate yourself and everyone around you who is succeeding. They are on their own path and have no competition with you or another. When you truly desire for everyone around you exactly what you desire for yourself the game changes. Abundance starts to flow towards you like you are a magnet for receiving. Make a commitment to yourself in your personal life, business, work & relations; don't take anything from anyone without giving them more & better. This is the success mantra that the universe wants you to know.

Give more than you can and you will receive more than you want.

Imagine walking in a beautiful garden with all kinds of flowers and leaves around you. What if this is exactly the world that you are passing through. Those flowers, leaves & thorns are people and experiences. Try to find your sacred source in everyone you meet and your energy will transcend to more compassionate loving energy. God is eternal bliss, infinite wisdom & intelligence, unconditional love, compassion, nirvana & ecstasy. When you find yourself in this state you have connected to your source energy very powerfully. Congratulations!

Your presence on this earth is very short. It's one of the journeys for your evolution. You have been blessed with infinite power inside you and moreover, you have your guides constantly around your aura. All you have to do is ask. Ask for guidance, ask for help, ask to be lead, and ask to be aligned, ask for direction. You will create, accomplish & achieve in a much magnified and correct manner when you involve the guidance of the masters & the 'Divine Intelligence' wisdom.

You have a powerful treasure inside you, the power of the 'Infinite Source Energy'; invoke that power to guide you for life.

Sacred Reminders
From Allah, Universe, Infinite Intelligence, Your Subconscious Mind, Your Eternal being

> *"How we see God is a direct reflection of how we see ourselves. If God brings to mind mostly fear and blame, it means there is too much fear and blame welled inside us. If we see God as full of love & compassion, so are we".*
>
> *—Elif Shafak (Rule #1 from 40 Rules of Love)*

NOV VII, MMXVIII

1. "I can neither be contained by my 'Earth' nor by my 'Skies'; but I can be contained by the 'Qulb' (soul) of a true believer. I am nearer to you than your jugular vein; don't look around for me anymore; look inside; Look into your soul; I'm there; closer than you thought imaginable; come reach me; and I'll be with you."

2. "Amongst 'MY' signs are the night and the day, and the sun and the moon. Night and day are opposites, and yet, by the alchemy, they can both sub serve the purpose of human good. The night gives rest while the day promotes activity. The sun and moon are similarly complimentary. So, in moral and spiritual affairs, seeming opposites may be made to sub serve the purposes of good."

3.   "Man does not weary of asking for good things. But if ill touches him, he gives up all hope and is lost in despair. I plan, guide, and control all things. To receive a little check; is to let you find your bearings and to let your thoughts turn to higher things."

4.   "The pursuit of happiness is detachment from this world, its attractions & relations. Be present and involved but always be detached; as the true life is hereafter. The lust of wealth and worldly power directs you to a temporary high. Peace comes from knowing that this life is just a journey towards the real life. There is happiness, sadness, loss, achievements, there is good and bad; all of this to test how you respond to MY calling."

5.   "The negative incidents in life are just a nudge to come back in MY embrace. In a way these moments, however painful are a redirection; for the better; if you believe."

6.   "Surrender; 'Let Go'; you will be amazed at the victory this will bring to you in every aspect of your being. EGO (NAFS) is a trap. As soon as you let go of your ego and surrender to the divine plan, your life will start to transform."

7.   "Three Relations are vital – Your relationship with your source, your relationship with yourself, and lastly your relationship with humanity."

8.   "Everything has a purpose. You are at your present stage through a variety of events, conditions & states. **Unto Thy LORD** is the ultimate goal of it. Your purpose is revealed to

you in moments. Keep your eyes open, your heart clear and your soul pure; your purpose will come to you in signs."

9.   "The success in life and beyond depends upon the amount of knowledge you acquire of the universe and upon the proper use of that knowledge. The success of the average soul is the achievement of wealth; whereas the real success is awareness & alignment with the wealth-giver."

10.   "Gratitude is key. If you are grateful I'll, give you more. Give endlessly & you will receive endlessly. Become the source rather than storage. Let it all flow through you; become a medium and you will be blessed forever."

11.   "Practice patience in adversity. Nothing is stagnant in this universe. Everything changes. This too shall pass; Trust me."

12.   "You are restless with a deep void inside. This void can never be filled with any worldly desire. You will achieve peace & serenity only by syncing yourself to the universe. That's your only source of peace. Everything else is unlimited chaos. Don't tire yourself."

13.   "And the lovers of the 'Most Beneficent' are those who walk on the earth in humility and sedateness, and when the foolish address them (with condescending words) they reply back with mild words of gentleness. Exude positivity & goodness; radiate nothing but good."

14.   "When My pure souls ask you about me, then (tell them that) I am near. Reach for me

inside your soul; I'm nearer to you than you can imagine."

15.   "It could be that you dislike something, when it is good for you; and it could be that you like something when it is bad for you. Surrender to MY plans as they happen. Adjust to the change. Go after your dreams with the flexibility of the course changes. They are for your benefit."

16.   "Ask, and It Shall Be Given To You". "Seek, and Ye Shall Find". "Knock, And It Shall Be Opened Unto You". "For Everyone that Asketh Receiveth."

The Golden Words

1.   Every thought, intention, choice, response & decision that you take in life either aligns you with your 'Worldly' aura or your 'Eternal' aura. Choose wisely.

2.   Ego or Love; every action or response that comes through you. Always ask yourself. Is it driven by my 'Ego' or 'Love'?

3.   Free your heart from desires. When you give up everything, you get everything.

4.   When you realize the truth that there is nothing lacking inside or around you; that's the exact moment when the entire world belongs to you.

5.   Accept the powers of the infinite intelligence, the divine source, and allow it to guide your life.

6.   Detachment; is key to gliding through this world, this temporary journey.

7.   Glide through this life; what comes in your experience let it come, what leaves your experience let it leave. Don't stagnate your heart for anything good or bad, keep gliding.

8.   Trust the universe's plan; learn to let go and go with the flow.

9.   Never follow money, fame, success, or people. Become the best version of yourself. All that you desire will flow towards you when you are ready.

10.   Dedicate your life to creating rather than competing.

11.   Learn to create and accomplish everything without getting attention. The universe creates and accomplishes everything everyday yet we don't hear a sound.

12.   Never close your heart due to negative worldly experiences; keep your heart open and flowing with love & light. Always.

13.   Understand your existence and your source and the meaning behind it. You are passing through this world as a temporary lesson, you have infinite divine intelligence inside you.

14.   The Universe is inside you. It is inexhaustible infinite divine energy inside your being. Tap into it and use it as much as you want. It is infinite.

15.   Identify your purpose and dedicate your life to it.

16.   Strive for respect not attention.

17.   Become a source of light & healing for humanity.

18.   Everything that you see is a reflection of 'God'. Eliminate the traits of hatred, jealousy, anger, resentment, negativity, judgment, vengeance, shame, cynicism & sadness from your heart & soul.

19.   Never stop learning & improving yourself. You are here in this world to learn, unlearn, know, experience & create. Use this time wisely.

20.   Be loving & kind to people who are good to you, be extra loving & kind to people who are not good to you.

21.   Every response that you initiate creates karma for you. When you respond with only love your karmic cycle tends to bring love to you in this life and after.

22.   Never force anything, never interfere with the universe events & experiences. Nothing happens without a reason. Understand this concept, accept, trust, let go & flow.

23.   This world is a temporary illusion. Your body is a cloak for this world only. Your source and your soul are eternal. Death is not negative; it's only a shift from one dimension to the other.

24.   Center yourself, ground yourself, and root yourself so strongly that nothing topples your being.

25.   Give up control, flow & glide to the universe's plan. Experience, learn & improve along your journey.

26.   Never desire another person's approval. You are a whole and an infinite being. You don't need approvals and validations. You are radiating perfect source light and you are striving for a fellow beings' approval?

27.   Adapt simplicity & humbleness in your aura. You will shine like a star.

28.   Never depend on money, success, fame, or another person for happiness, fulfillment & contentment. These traits are satisfied only by your own infinite source energy.

29.   Contrast is the essence of this temporary world. The good comes with the bad and the negative comes with the positive. Darkness & light, happiness & sadness are inseparable so if

you desire or experience one you have to experience another. That's the law of this earth energy. The key is to learn how to be stable in both experiences. No need for excessive celebration in elation and no use of excessive sadness in adversity.

30.   Change is the only constant. Don't cling to anyone or anything as everything is in motion and proceeding to change. Nothing stays the same as per law of this universe.

31.   Adapt the traits of water. Be so transparent & clear that light radiates from you, be so soft that you mold yourself to all the transitions in your life, be so hard that you can cut through the rocks of pain.

32.   We are all linked energy in this world. We are all a part of each other. Nothing is separate. The good and the evil are part of us.

33.   It is not how much you do but how well you do things. Work smarter not harder.

34.   Learn the 'Art of Flow' and instill the concept of gliding through life without attaching ourselves to anything good or bad.

35.   Adapt the traits of the 'Divine Source Power'. Be available to humanity, yet unreachable. Rise above the worldly desires & events.

36.   You are human and you will make mistakes during your learning journey. The wise soul acknowledges the mistakes, accepts and corrects faults, learns from them, and improves constantly.

37.   You are human and you will experience & feel all emotions. The art of living is to acknowledge & accept these emotions, feel them, and detach yourself. Don't stay there for too long. They will cling to your being and drown you into worldly sadness, depression, negativity & pessimism.

38.   Pain, failure, negativity, hurt & experiences like death & loss that shake you to your core are all lessons for you. They are opportunities in disguise for your growth.

39.   Death is inevitable; soul is eternal. The ones you lose to death are in a better place, their test is over.

40.   Any loss is painful yet has a purpose. Contemplate through this experience to learn. Sometimes the universe removes people from your life as they can't go to the level that you have to go. Sometimes you lose people because your vibrations are lower than where they have to rise. The universe knows best.

41.   Pain & happiness both are inevitable, yet detach yourself from both as each will be followed by the contrast eventually.

42.   You are here in this world to create not compete. There is no competition with anyone.

43.   Your creation must benefit humanity. Create & give; the two powerful traits.

44.   Cherish & honor happiness around you, your family, your loved ones, mother earth, your purpose, and devote your life to this.

45.   Walk on earth; yes, walk barefoot on grass, touch a tree, talk to plants, as these will

center and ground you. We are surrounded by electronics and lower frequency auras and activities. Ground yourself often to neutralize the negative effects of all this and sync back to mother earth frequency as often as possible.

46. The more you give the more you get; simple law of universe. Now go and give exactly what you want in your life in abundance.

47. Fill your heart with the treasures of the divine power, compassion, love, humility & patience.

48. Be so humble that nothing and no one feels better than you. You are not superior to anyone or anything. Just align to your source and be.

49. Center & ground yourself so much that no praise elates you and no negativity or criticism discourages you.

50. Simplicity is the ultimate power. Simplify your life, your living, your desires, your world, your home, yourself.

51. Adopt the minimalistic approach. Instead of finding happiness in accumulating possessions, open your heart & hands and give. Give love, care, food, money to the needy, and give your time. This is where true happiness resides.

52. Blaming someone else is a cowardly trait; rise above it. You are where you are because of your previous dimension karmic lessons, your choices, acceptances, and manifestations of your thoughts throughout your life. You want better experiences, improve your thoughts & actions.

53.   Analyze yourself constantly. You are not perfect. You are learning till your last breath. Your source is perfect and once you learn how to tap into your source and align yourself with it, you will become the universe.

54.   We are all here on this earth going through lessons & karmic experiences. You will see happiness & grief, you will see evil & good, and you will experience pain & joy. Let it be. Don't judge, blame, or hate anything. Everyone you see including yourself is going through a journey that started with their soul many dimensions back. We are all experiencing our karmic lessons. We are all balancing the good & bad we have chosen and experienced in our previous dimensions.

55.   'God', 'The Universe', and our 'Divine Source' is not cruel. It's just letting us be. We are experiencing results of our own choices from this world dimension and many dimensions before. If you want a different result improve your thoughts, raise your vibration, and make better choices.

56.   Every emotion you feel is a message from your soul. Analyze your emotions & find their root. Heal yourself accordingly

57.   Gratitude is trusting the universe. Be thankful at the end of each day for everything.

58.   For anything that troubles your heart; just say to the universe that I'd like to see the highest possible outcome.

59.   In life, in business, in work, in relationships, in all aspects of your being, leave

someone with more than you take from them. When you keep the weight of giving heavier on your end you always attract a hundred times more. The honor is in being a source of giving.

60.   You are a 'Timeless soul' in a 'Timed world'. Use this short duration on earth wisely to learn, align & evolve for your highest good.

61.   When you trust the 'Divine Intelligence' for guidance and direction, you automatically choose the highest outcome. When you make a choice yourself, you override the divine wisdom as it doesn't have power over your choice. It guides you but ultimately your choice determines the outcome.

62.   If you are constantly attracting negativity or painful experiences, analyze your thoughts, your intentions, your choices, your vibrations. You attract at the frequency that you are. Elevate & Improve.

63.   Your subconscious mind is not working against your conscious mind. The power is to align & unite both these minds; keeping a balance amongst them.

64.   Focus and attract only those who are in harmony and alignment with your current intentions and vibrations. Surround yourself by souls who desire vibrational elevation, positivity, growth, and help others.

65.   Rejoice in other's happiness and prosperity. Never condemn another's success, abundance, or wealth. That is a destined formula to condemn the same for yourself as karma is surely one of the spiritual laws.

66.   The idea is not to 'Achieve' but 'Align'. Once you align, everything will automatically fall into place bringing you peace, serenity, abundance & success.

67.   People around you are your actual test on this 'Earth Journey'. You will be tested through them; through the relations.

68.   The universe has another secret law; 'Law of Direction'. Every moment of your life there is a direction for the next; only if you listen closely.

69.   Night is only the absence of sunlight. Evil is nothing but an absence of Divine Light. Become the divine light.

70.   Your 'Life Mantra' now: 'ALIGN, ASK & ALLOW.'

Kun Fayakun
Be & It is

Kun Fayakun; an Arabic phrase that appears in the Quran. 'Kun' means 'to exist' and 'to be'; whereas 'Fayakun means 'It is". Together this phrase is the Almighty's power that translates as **"Be & It is"**.

When the Almighty, the Eternal Entity allows; it manifests. Chant "Kun Fayakun" in your meditation and by the power of the 'Infinite Source' your dreams manifest to reality.

Fana Baqa

(The process of surrender & EGO (Nafs) Elimination)

"Fana' is the annihilation of self; the ego (nafs) & "Baqa" is rising from that surrendered state back to reality as a re-birth. A genesis in the same world but an evolved and changed self. A journey to self-awareness & finding our purpose. 'Fana" is the state of dissolving our being to the frequency of the Eternal Entity.

Ego (nafs) is the culprit of most of our actions, reactions & choices. It is always choosing between intellect, wisdom & desire. Dissolving the ego purifies our soul, raises our vibration, and opens us up to the universe beyond the worldly dimension.

TawakkuL

(God Consciousness)

'Tawakkul" is 'Trust' in the Almighty/ Universe's plan, yet doing our part in the worldly realm. It's the unwavering belief with commitment & effort.

It's the secret for the 'Timed World' & the 'Timeless Eternity'

Affirmation

I am ready to receive the message. I allow myself to receive the wisdom, guidance, knowledge, direction & Faith that the universe is sending to me through the words in this book and many more books like this. I am ready, I allow and my healing and transformation begins now!

Inspirations & References

This book is a personal research-based entity and has no link whatsoever with anyone or any corporation. The words are from the research conducted by me, author 'Amber Khan' personally over the course of two decades. Reference quotes from different books are added with the book title or the author's name for credit and reference. This is a spiritual book meant to heal souls and raise vibrations in the spiritual realm of this universe. Research done for this book is based on books, online search engines, encyclopedia, and Holy books. Holding credit for my own writing and honoring with gratitude the writings of my spiritual gurus. The knowledge attained and expressed is inspired from treasures of;

- *The Quran*
- *The Bible*
- *Tripitaka*

Spiritual Teachers, Mentors, Poets, Philosophers & Authors who consistently inspired & influence my writings are;

- *The Prophet Mohammad SAW*
- *Hazrat Bibi Rabia Basri*
- *Shams Tabrizi*
- *Mevlana Jalaludin RUMI*
- *Shykh Hakim Moinuddin Chishti*
- *Bulle Shah*
- *Khalil Jibran (Kahlil Jibran)*

- *Dalai Lama*
- *Dr. Allama Iqbal*
- *Qudrat Ullah Shahab*
- *Syed Ali bin Uthman Al-Hujweri*
- *Thich Nhat Hanh*
- *Carl Jung*
- *Sigmund Freud*
- *William Shakespeare*
- *Dr. Andrew Weil*
- *Elif Shafak*
- *Paulo Coelho*
- *Marcus Aurelius*
- *Napoleon Hill*
- *Gary Zukav*
- *Osho*
- *Mantak Chia*
- *Ram Dass*
- *Pema Chodron*
- *Dr. Wayne Dyer*
- *Eckhart Tolle*
- *Viktor E. Frankl*
- *Robert Greene*
- *Earl Nightingale*
- *Wallace D Wattles*
- *Annie Besant*
- *Uell S. Anderson*
- *Thomson Jay Hudson*
- *Thomas Troward*
- *Sun Tzu*
- *Dr. Sebi*
- *Og Mandino*

- *Dale Carnegie*
- *Nassim Nicholas Taleb*
- *Mark Victor Hansen*
- *Robert Allen*
- *Imam Ibne Qayim*
- *Karen Armstrong*
- *Allan Watts*
- *Mitch Albom*
- *Pam Grout*
- *Jane Roberts*
- *Esther Hicks*
- *Zig Ziglar*
- *Mark Twain*
- *Oscar Wilde*
- *F. Scott Fitzgerald*
- *Stephen Covey*
- *Robert Kiyosaki*
- *Robin S. Sharma*
- *Deepak Chopra*
- *Hal Elrod*
- *Satchin Panda*
- *Joseph Murphy*
- *J. Krishnamurti*
- *Donald Robertson*
- *Michael A. Singer*
- *Marianne Williamson*
- *Norman Vincent Peale*
- *Sabrina Reber*
- *Subroto Bagchi*
- *Yasmin Mogahed*

I would highly recommend everyone on the journey of transition, healing & spirituality to read these valuable authors & spiritual masters.

**Research platforms: Wikipedia, Thesaurus & images courtesy Shutterstock.*

Book Writing Dates

October 29, 2012 (Scottsdale)

January 2, 2013, (Lahore)

May 31, 2013 (Koh Samui)

October 17, 2013 (Lahore)

April 5, 2014 (Islamabad)

July 26, 2014 (Lahore)

October 25, 2014 (Sedona)

December 7, 2014 (Sedona)

June 28, 2015 (Istanbul)

March 26, 2017 (Konya)

September 10, 2017 (Istanbul)

February 27, 2019 (Austin)

July 7, 2019 (Tbilisi)

July 13, 2019 (Baku)

August 13, 2019 (Austin)

November 21, 2019 (Istanbul) and March 2020 (Lahore)

About Author

Amber Khan; a Sufi soul, a painter, writer, motivational speaker & 'Holistic/High Vibrational Lifestyle' practitioner & teacher. Empowering souls to transform their lives, heal & align them with their gift; their purpose. Teaching compassion with unconditional love creating a ripple effect in the world for more love and peace.

For feedback, Reviews & Comments please email: amber@nureamber.com

---

You are a 'Timeless soul' in a 'Timed world'.

You are not here on this earth to suffer, you are here to flow, learn, create, ascend, assist, and connect to your source.

Reviews

"This ought to be required reading for those on the 'Path of Transformation' into their true selves. Magical read. It made me change the way I think and opened up my eyes to different perspectives. It shook my soul. I learnt how to converse with the Universe without hesitation. I thought I already knew how to do this through meditation but the words in this book uncover something that I just can't explain. You can feel the kind and loving intent within every word. This book is very easy to read and understand; you really don't need advanced philosophy to move mountains of the mind. What a gift, what a treasure. "A. Wali

"Very powerful, well-written and informative" Zaimah K.

www.ingramcontent.com/pod-product-compliance
Lightning Source LLC
Chambersburg PA
CBHW031054250726
48655CB00004B/1429